2004

Well and Good

Well and Good:
a case study approach to biomedical ethics

third edition

John E. Thomas and Wilfrid J. Waluchow

broadview press

Canadian Cataloguing in Publication Data
Thomas, John E., 1926-1996
    Well and good: a case study approach to biomedical ethics

3rd ed.
Includes bibliographical references and index.
ISBN 1-55111-206-X
1. Medical ethics - Case studies.   2. Bioethics - Case studies.
I. Waluchow, Wilfrid J., 1953- .   II. Title.
R724.T48 1998   174'.2   C98-930793-X

Broadview Press Ltd., is an independent, international publishing house, incorporated in 1985.

North America:
P.O. Box 1243, Peterborough, Ontario, Canada K9J 7H5
3576 California Road, Orchard Park, NY 14127
TEL: (705) 743-8990; FAX: (705) 743-8353;
E-MAIL: customerservice@broadviewpress.com

United Kingdom:
Turpin Distribution Services Ltd.,
Blackhorse Rd., Letchworth, Hertfordshire SG6 1HN
TEL: (1462) 672555; FAX (1462) 480947; E-MAIL: turpin@rsc.org

Australia:
St. Clair Press, P.O. Box 287, Rozelle, NSW 2039
TEL: (02) 818-1942; FAX: (02) 418-1923

www.broadviewpress.com

Broadview Press gratefully acknowledges the support of the Ontario Arts Council, and the Ministry of Canadian Heritage. We acknowledge the financial support of the Government of Canada through the Book Publishing Industry Development Program for our publishing activities.

Text design and composition by George Kirkpatrick

PRINTED IN CANADA

For Mo and John
As loving a couple as ever there was.

Contents

Preface to the Third Edition

At the time of his death in October of 1996, John Thomas and I had just begun working on the third edition of *Well and Good*. New cases were in the works, as was an expanded version of our introductory chapter on ethical theory. With the encouragement and assistance of John's wife, Mo, I took it upon myself to complete the job John and I had begun. The new edition contains an expanded section of unanalyzed cases, covering topics such as jumping the queue in the OR, fetal sex selection for non-medical reasons, and the responsibilities of critical care nurses. In addition, four new analyzed cases have been added: Sue Rodriguez and her claim to physician-assisted suicide; the tragic "mercy-killing" of Tracy Latimer by her father, Robert; the case of Ms. G., the glue-sniffing, expectant mother; and material on the Canadian "tainted blood scandal." The introduction to ethical theory now includes sections on Aristotle's "virtue ethics" and "feminist bioethics." Finally, many of the analyzed cases which remain from the second edition have been updated in light of new developments and the expanded section on ethical theory.

Completing this edition of *Well and Good* was difficult without the help and encouragement of my co-author. The heavy burden was lightened, however, by the invaluable assistance of our wives and best friends, Donna Waluchow and Mo Thomas. Many thanks to them both.

Wil Waluchow
McMaster University

Acknowledgements

We wish to acknowledge the contributions and valuable assistance of the following colleagues in compiling and modifying some of the cases contained in this volume, the majority of which are Canadian in origin. Unless otherwise indicated those listed below are members of the Faculty of Health Sciences, McMaster University.

Dr. William Scott Beattie, Professor of Anaesthesiology
Dr. David Carr, Professor of Anatomy
Dr. R. Davidson, Professor Emeritus of Pediatrics and Pathology
Ms. Sandra Dawson, Department of Philosophy, McMaster University
Dr. P.B. Dent, Professor and Chairman, Pediatrics
Dr. Bernard M. Dickens, Faculty of Law, University of Toronto
Ms. Jaimie Dianda, Genetics Associate
Dr. John Hay, Emeritus Professor of Family Medicine
Dr. D.L. Hitchcock, Department of Philosophy, McMaster University
Dr. John Jarrell, Professor of Obstetrics and Gynecology, Foothills Hospital, Calgary
Dr. A.L. Johnson, Emeritus Professor of Clinical Epidemiology and Biostatistics
Dr. P. Knight, Professor of Surgery
Dr. C.B. Mueller, Emeritus Professor of Surgery
Dr. Jennifer Parks, Department of Philosophy, Loyola University, Chicago
Dr. J.C. Sinclair, Professor of Pediatrics
Dr. J. Soni, Psychiatry, Hamilton Psychiatric Hospital
Dr. D.L. Streiner, Professor of Clinical Epidemiology and Biostatistics
Mr. R.C. Walker, President, Faculty of Health Sciences
Dr. J.L. Watts, Professor of Pediatrics
Dr. Michael Yeo, Bioethicist, Canadian Medical Association

Much of the work on the first edition of this book was made possible by a McMaster University Teaching and Learning Grant. This, too, is gratefully acknowledged.

Finally, we express our deep appreciation to Mo for her support, help, and unfailing patience.

Introduction: Ethical Resources for Decision-Making

(1) Moral Philosophy

Decision-making in medicine has always had a moral dimension. The current prominence enjoyed by biomedical ethics is due, in no small measure, to the impact of biochemistry and improved technology. There is much more that can be done for (or to) patients than could ever be done before. New technological possibilities raise all sorts of questions which never had to be faced in the past. At one time the question "What *should* be done?" may have been more or less equivalent to the question "What *can* be done?" Whether or not this was true in the past, it is clearly not true now. To take one example: medicine is now able to keep people alive on respirators and other life-support mechanisms in situations where many question the propriety of doing so. If someone is irreversibly comatose, it may be that we *can* keep her alive. But whether we *should* utilize scarce resources to do so is another question altogether. So ethics plays an extremely important role in the practice of medicine.

What are the respective roles to be played by health-care professionals on the one hand, and moral philosophers or "ethicists" on the other? Moral philosophers are not moral experts capable of providing ready-made answers when difficult or intransigent moral conflicts arise in medicine. Rather, they perform more modest tasks: clarifying the terms of moral debate, scrutinizing distinctions to see if they stand up to rational examination, assessing the validity and cogency of arguments, and examining the fit between moral practice and moral principles and values.

Moral philosophers are of course also concerned sometimes with defending their own moral theories and convictions, particularly when they detect unwarranted, dogmatic beliefs. But a student unaccustomed to the ways of the moral philosopher will often find the philosopher's arguments a trifle strange. The moral philosopher will often seek to defend or justify the obvious – e.g., that it is morally wrong intentionally to deceive a patient about the dangerous side-effects of an experimental drug the patient is being asked to take, or that it is wrong deliberately to enrol mentally competent patients in clinical trials without their consent. At other times, the moral philosopher will offer arguments which *question* the obvious. She might even try to defend a position which strikes others as patently false – e.g., that elderly people have less right to scarce medical resources than younger people. The main reason for these strange activities of the moral philosopher lies in his chief motivation, expressed in a maxim propounded by the ancient Greek philosopher Socrates. According to Socrates, the unexamined life is not worth living. Socrates and other moral philosophers always want to know *why* we should believe the things we do, even those things which we firmly and passionately believe to be true. Many of our moral beliefs just seem right to us. We've never had occasion to question them or to ask ourselves why we hold them. Yet if pushed to articulate the grounds or bases of our moral beliefs, we are often unable to provide them. And even if we do manage to come up with something, we often find that our grounds do not stand up well to critical scrutiny. It may seem obvious that no patient should be enroled in a clinical drug trial without the prior consent of the patient or a person entitled to give consent on the patient's behalf. This principle, P, helps to explain why we would condemn a physician/experimenter who, without first gaining informed consent, tried out a new drug on a group of patients in their thirties who had lung cancer but were otherwise normal adults.

But now ask whether principle P stands up to rational scrutiny. Imagine that you are on an Ethics Review Board at a University Hospital and that a project in which principle P seems to be compromised comes before the Board for approval. The situation is as follows.

Babies are sometimes born with a hypotensive condition for which potentially life-saving medication is immediately required. Your hospital has routinely used two types of medication to combat this condition, some physicians preferring the one drug, X, others the second, Y. Both X and Y seem effective, but they operate in different ways. It is also unclear whether X or Y is preferable in terms of degree of efficacy or severity of potential side-effects. The doctors want to clear up these uncertainties and ascertain whether X or Y is better. A trial is proposed in which all new-born babies with hypotension will be randomly allocated to receive either X or Y. The study protocol calls for "double blinding." That is, no one, including the doctors and nurses in the neonatal ward who will be administering the medication, will know to which group any particular baby has been assigned. There is only one hitch. Hypotension is not a condition which can be predicted before birth. Therefore it is not feasible to gain consent from parents before their baby is born. It is also not feasible, in most cases, to gain consent after birth when it becomes apparent that medication for hypotension is immediately required. As a consequence, the researcher suggests the following. If the parents are available, they will be asked to consent to enrolment of their baby in the study. If they object, their baby will then receive whichever of X or Y the attending physician happens to prefer. If they consent to their baby's participation, then the baby will be enroled in the study and assigned, randomly and blindly, either to the group receiving X or to the group receiving Y. As for those babies whose parents are unavailable when the necessity for immediate medication becomes apparent, they will be enroled in the study *without consent*. The parents of these babies will be contacted, however, as soon as possible and asked for consent to the continued enrolment of their baby. Should there be any objections at this stage, the choice of the baby's medication will then fall into the hands of the attending physician who will exercise his discretion in choosing X or Y.

Given that both X and Y are standard drugs in common use at the hospital, that parents are given the choice of opting out as soon as they can be reached, and that the proposed procedure for gaining consent is the only feasible one under the circumstances, it seems reasonable, and ethical, to permit temporary enrolment in the study without the parents' consent. But then doesn't this show that principle P must be rejected, or at least modified in some way? If so, what might the alternative be? We need to develop a moral theory for distinguishing cases where *prior* consent is vital from special cases in which it may not be necessary. It is here that the moral philosopher might be of some help. He might be able to supply an ethical theory upon the basis of which it is possible to support a reasonable alternative to P.

The family of activities pursued by the moral philosopher is prompted largely by a desire for clarity of thought and integrity of action – by Socrates's maxim that the unexamined life is not worth living. The student of moral philosophy must be prepared to approach the subject with the correct frame of mind, with a willingness to challenge the obvious and to consider seriously both the questionable and the unfamiliar. Should she do so, there is much of value that can be gleaned from the study of biomedical ethics.

One final point about the role of the moral philosopher. Moral philosophy is not the moral conscience of medicine and the related professions. On the contrary, moral philosophers should be viewed as partners with health-care professionals in worrying through troublesome moral questions which arise in the controversial territory where technical skills converge with human values. Moral philosophers are not out simply to criticize for moral failure – except perhaps when blind dogma rules moral practice, where the lives we lead do remain largely unexamined. Most important of all, perhaps, is the following point. To raise or consider moral questions surrounding biomedical practice is not necessarily to imply that there is something inherently immoral or unethical about what is going on. Nor is it to question the integrity of health-care professionals. The questions which arise in biomedical practice are difficult ones, and those who disagree with us or are generally perplexed do not necessarily have any less moral integrity than we do.

(2) Morality Versus Ethics

Moral persons are equally distributed in all walks of life, including medicine. Health-care professionals agonize over what is the right thing to do in difficult cases, and for the most part succeed in doing it. This is true whether the issue is withholding the truth from a terminally ill patient or using fetal tissue to help victims of Parkinson's Disease. As noted earlier, morality is always of relevance in medicine, and no one can claim to be a moral expert. Ethics or ethical theory is another matter. Ethical theory, as opposed to morality, is the systematic, critical study of the basic underlying principles, values, and concepts utilized in thinking about moral life. Ethics, so understood, is something the average person concerns himself with only infrequently, if ever. But this is not true of moral philosophers or ethicists. They are primarily concerned with ethical theory. They have developed concepts, theories, and techniques of argument which can often be of use to non-philosophers in finding their way through the tangled moral issues to which the practice of medicine often gives rise. We would do well, then, to consider the general ethical theories of some of the most influential moral philosophers of Western civilization. This we will do in later sections. First, a few thoughts on the nature and role of ethical theories.

(3) Levels of Moral Response

Consider the question "Why do you oppose abortion?" As put to an opponent of abortion, this question can trigger different types of responses.

(a) The Expressive Level

At the most primitive level the answer is likely to be: "Because abortion is repugnant" or "I hate the very thought of killing a fetus." These responses are unanalyzed expressions or feelings which, in themselves, do not constitute any kind of justification or reason for opposing abortion. This is not to deny that feelings are relevant to morality or that moral convictions are often accompanied by strong emotions. It is simply to say that the mere fact that one feels a certain way about an action or practice in no way constitutes an adequate justification for making moral pronouncements on it.

(b) The Pre-reflective Level

At the next level of response, justification is offered by reference to values, rules, and principles – i.e., norms – accepted uncritically. Most often it is offered by reference to what we will call, somewhat loosely, a "conventional" norm. Such a standard may be expressed in a legal rule, in one of society's conventionally accepted values, in a religious pronouncement, or in a professional code of ethics. At this level of response one's opposition to abortion might take the following form: "I disapprove of abortion because my priest informs me that it is morally wrong" or "I disapprove of treating patients without their consent because this is prohibited by the professional code governing my national Medical Association."

It is a defining feature of the pre-reflective level of response that its conventional norms are uncritically accepted and acted upon. We don't stop to think why we should act or base our judgments upon the conventional norms or if they are good standards to adopt. Assuming that the conventional norms are good ones, any ensuing behaviour may be classified as conventionally moral or ethical, but it is important to realize that it is a species of externally directed behaviour. It is the blind following of standards or norms set by someone else. As noted, this is not necessarily bad. Sometimes conventional norms are capable of reasoned defence and can be fully justified morally. Sometimes there is even good moral reason to follow conventional rules just because they are conventionally accepted. Conventional norms can help to foster common understandings and serve to ground justified expectations in others concerning how we will conduct ourselves. Sometimes it is crucial to know that other people will be playing by the same rules that we are. Imagine what it would be like if there were no conventionally agreed rules governing the making of promises. We would never be certain whether a promise had been made or whether its author considered it binding.

It is a serious mistake, however, to think that morality is exhausted by conventional norms alone or that moral justification *ends* with the invocation of a conventional rule. The norms must always be subject to critical moral scrutiny. Perhaps there are much better rules which we should try to persuade others to adopt. Or perhaps existing conventions are morally objectionable. That X is generally accepted as morally right never, in itself, entails that X is morally right. Slavery was at one time widely accepted as morally correct. Slavery was, and always will be, morally wrong nonetheless. It is quite possible that practices currently sanctioned by conventional morality should likewise be modified or rejected. Morality requires eternal vigilance: we must always think about the justification of what we are about to do, or at least be prepared always to do so.

(c) The Reflective Level
At this level of response our moral judgments are not based entirely on conventional norms blindly accepted, but on principles, rules and values to which we ourselves consciously subscribe and with regard to which we, as rational moral agents, are prepared to offer reasoned moral defence. It is possible of course that the norms to which we subscribe at the reflective level are in fact norms conventionally accepted as well. They might, for instance, be those which have found their way into a professional code (e.g. the AMA or CMA Codes of Ethics) by which one is expected to abide. The point is that at the reflective level of moral response we must be prepared to consider questions of justification. We must not blindly accept the conventional norms but be

prepared to consider for ourselves whether they are justified, or whether other, perhaps wholly novel, norms are those by which people should lead their lives.

At the reflective level, opposition to abortion may now take the form: "I oppose abortion because the fetus's right to life takes precedence over the woman's right to control her own reproductive processes." Here a reason is given – a basis or ground for the moral judgment is provided. The complexity and sophistication of the reflective level of response is evident from the presence of competing judgments and the plausible bases for them. One can imagine, as a reply to the above, the following retort: "Abortion is morally permissible because the rights of *actual* persons (pregnant women) take precedence over the rights of *potential* persons (fetuses)." As this example illustrates, ethics at the reflective level admits of few easy answers!

Of the three levels considered, the reflective level is the one at which most of the discussion in the present book takes place. This is so despite grounds for misgivings about the possibilities for full resolution of moral controversies at the reflective level. Reflection does not guarantee agreement. As will be evident throughout this book, moral reflection often yields only "a" but not "the only" defensible position. Not only do people feel differently at the expressive level, and uncritically favour different conventional rules at the pre-reflective level, they also often reach different conclusions at the reflective level. It is important to stress, once again, that there are no moral experts and that at each level, including the reflective one, we are often met with genuine dilemmas and competing bases for moral belief. Arriving at unassailable moral judgments is difficult, and some think impossible, not only because there are different levels of moral response, but also because people approach moral questions with very different perspectives.

(4) A Variety of Perspectives

The different approaches that moral agents take to moral questions may be illustrated by distinguishing between three ways in which the term "know" can be used.

(i) Sometimes the claim to know amounts to nothing more than a claim to feel sure or certain. This yields no more than a subjective, psychological criterion. While emotionally reassuring, a feeling of certainty is not a reliable mark of bona fide moral judgments. Others with different, even opposing, moral views may feel just as strongly that they are right. One who claims to know, and tries to add as a warrant that he just feels certain about what he believes, offers no warrant at all. His certainty is no more a warrant than the certainty with which many people at one time believed slavery to be morally justified.

(ii) Next the claim to know may be reduced to: "The position I hold is the one for which the best reasoned justification seems possible." Such a claim acknowledges the requirement of reasoned defence and that the position held may not be the only defensible one. It recognizes that rational people of good will and integrity may reasonably disagree about moral matters and that no one can claim, with absolute certainty, to have *the right* answer.

(iii) The third use of "know" is much stronger than the second and, according to many moral philosophers, quite unwarranted. It is equivalent to: "I know my view is the right one, and anyone who disagrees with me suffers from moral blindness, error or misunderstanding." Leaving aside the question of whether, in moral life, there are ever uniquely correct solutions to moral issues, the degree of self-assurance echoed in the above claim amounts to sheer audacity and arrogance. Even a commitment to the notion that there is "a final truth" in ethics should be accompanied by the acknowledgement that in practice we must often operate in humility with only partial knowledge and approximations to the truth. Moral progress is possible at both the social and the personal levels. Just as we believe that a society's practices can improve morally, as when America abandoned slavery, we should always believe that our own personal practices and beliefs can be improved, usually by listening to what others, whose opinions we respect, have to say.

Misgivings about the ethical enterprise may go even deeper than the foregoing comments suggest. There are profound philosophical disputes about the status of ethics itself – about whether moral judgments are in the end capable of full justification. Three of the more extreme difficulties are as follows.

(a) The Issue of Verification
The problem of verification in the context of moral judgments may

be illustrated by reference to the following scenario. Apple Mary is sitting in the downtown Hamilton market selling her produce. Suddenly a furtive-looking character sneaks up behind her and clubs her. As she falls to the ground, her assailant scoops up her purse and vanishes.

Imagine two witnesses commenting as follows:

A. Did you see that?
B. I did.
A. What a dreadful thing to happen in our town.
B. I agree.
A. What that man did was terribly wrong.
B. I didn't see anything wrong.
A. How can you possibly say that?
B. Easily. Let's go over carefully what happened.
A. Let's do that.
B. I saw Apple Mary sitting at her stall. I saw a man creep up behind her. I saw him lift a club and bring it down on her head. I saw Mary slump to the ground and her assailant take off with her purse. I didn't see any wrong.

The clue to the dispute between A and B is to be found in the ambiguity of the word "see." Of course B is correct if by "see" we mean physical seeing. We do not see the wrong in the way we see arms raised, clubs wielded, and purses snatched. Moral seeing is more like "seeing that" (making a judgment) than seeing with our eyes. We see *that* assault is wrong. We see *that* stealing is wrong. Moral insights are expressed in the form of judgments which are not verifiable empirically in the way that observational statements are. Rather they are substantiated by reference to principles, rules, or values which serve as their ground or warrant. According to the first ethical theory we will examine, as well as one version of the second, we justify our actions in terms of the following schemata:

$$\text{principles}$$
$$\downarrow$$
$$\text{rules}$$
$$\downarrow$$
$$\text{actions or judgments}$$

The contemplated action, or a moral judgment concerning it, falls under a rule, and the rule, in turn, conforms to a higher-order principle. By contrast, the third routine we will consider involves identifying principles specifying "prima facie duties," and in situations of conflicting prima facie duties, determining which takes precedence. But more on this later. The point to be stressed at this stage is that we do not see moral properties in the way we see the club which hit Apple Mary. Moral judgments are not open to empirical verification – indeed, they cannot be substantiated by way of a universally agreed routine or procedure. There are a plurality of competing theories on how our moral judgments are to be substantiated. Most, but not all, may be mapped onto the above schemata.

(b) A Plurality of Ethical Systems

The existence of a plurality of different approaches to the justification of moral judgments may be a cause for dismay. It is one thing to be made aware that the morality of our actions is not open to empirical verification; it is quite another to learn that different ethical theories prescribe quite different routines to be utilized in moral reasoning. It would certainly be simpler if there were only one theory and one routine. The only problems then remaining would be problems of casuistry (i.e. application of rules or principles to particular cases). But philosophers have yet to discover an ethical theory upon which all reasonable people agree, and as we have already seen, there are those who believe that no such theory will ever be found. As the understanding we have of ourselves and the world around us increases, we should expect our ethical theories to change, and we hope, progress. In this particular respect, ethics is no different from science where change and progress are routinely accepted as inevitable. The best we can do at present is to engage in the pursuit of a defensible ethical theory and try to learn as much as we can from those who have done so in the past. There is much to be learned from the theorists whose views will be outlined below.

(c) The Limits of Justification

If one were to adopt, for example, a Kantian or rule-utilitarian position, the prescribed routine for justifying moral judgments would be more or less clear. It might be difficult to tell precisely what action the theory required of us in a particular case, but it would be reasonably clear how to go about trying to answer that question. For Kant, as we shall see, an action is morally obligatory if it conforms to a rule and the rule, in turn, conforms to a principle which Kant calls the Categorical Imperative. For a rule-utilitarian there is an analogous procedure. Our actions must conform to a rule, and the rule must conform not to the Categorical Imperative but to the principle of utility. For fully committed utilitarians or Kantians, justification is limited to judgments made within the prescribed framework. We inquire, "Does the action in question conform to the rule and the rule to the (appropriate) principle?" If the answer is affirmative, the morality of the action is settled and we know what the theory prescribes as the right thing to do.

It is possible, of course, for a rule-utilitarian to raise questions about Kant's Categorical Imperative or for a Kantian to challenge the principle of utility. This involves raising questions concerning the validity of the frameworks themselves. In such cases what we have is a deeply philosophical dispute, the kind of dispute which is a primary concern of ethical theorists. Utilitarians and Kantians will marshal philosophical arguments which challenge the validity of the other's ethical theory. They will do so even when it is clear what actions the opposing frameworks require of us in particular cases, or even when the different frameworks prescribe exactly the same actions. The two theorists may agree on *what* we should do but disagree about *why* we should do it. Again, the reason is clear: the philosopher is concerned to understand why we should do certain things and refrain from doing others.

External philosophical questions concerning the validity of ethical frameworks are best dealt with in books devoted exclusively to ethical theory. This is not such a book. In what follows we shall outline five competing frameworks and only briefly mention some of the many external, philosophical questions which have been raised about them. Some students will likely feel a strong affinity for one of the five theories discussed below, but most will find something of value in each one. This is not surprising. Four of the theories to be examined reflect currents of thought which have dominated western culture in recent centuries, and the fifth is expressive of a powerful contemporary movement of thought. For those strongly inclined to think that one of the theories represents the truth of the matter, the old adage should be borne in mind: "Those who live in glass houses should not throw stones." External challenges to other systems should be seasoned with a measure of caution and humility and the recognition that questions of morality and ethics are ones upon which reasonable people of good will and integrity do often disagree.

They should also be informed by the wisdom of John Stuart Mill's observation that "conflicting doctrines, instead of one being true and the other false, [often] share the truth between them, and the nonconforming opinion is needed to supply the remainder of the truth of which the received doctrine embodies only a part."[1]

Given these profound difficulties with the ethical enterprise, the student may wonder why we should bother at all with an introduction to ethical theory. Why not just get on with an analysis of the various specific, moral issues that arise in the practice of health care, issues like prescribing birth control pills to minors or screening fetuses for genetic defects? One response is that we are not warranted in dropping ethical theory altogether simply because it has difficulties. Quantum physics is fraught with theoretical difficulties too, but it would be silly to give it up entirely because of this. Another response is that there are valuable lessons to be learned from the ways in which some of the greatest thinkers within our cultural history have seriously and systematically approached ethical issues. These are thinkers whose formulations have been extremely influential and whose theories provide the frameworks within which current ethical disputes are argued. One cannot get too far in modern moral debate without encountering some appeal to the concept of utility or to the value of individual autonomy. These concepts are the cornerstones of the theories of Mill and Kant respectively.

(5) Some Basic Concepts

Before turning to examine the theories of Kant, Mill, Ross, Aristotle, and the feminists, let us consider some basic terminology that is employed by ethical theorists. This terminology will be introduced by way of noting several distinctions.

First we should distinguish between *judgments of obligation* and *judgments of value*. Judgments of obligation concern what we ought to do. In expressing such judgments, we use sentences like: "You *ought* to take all steps to save human life"; "Your overriding *duty* was to protect the interests of your patient, not her fetus"; "You were under an obligation to honour your patient's wishes"; "It wasn't right to proceed without consent"; "He had a right to your best clinical judgment." All these judgments have to do directly with our conduct, with how we should behave.

Judgments of value, by contrast, are not directly related to action. These are judgments not about the right thing to do but about what is *good* or has *value*. For instance the judgments that freedom is a good thing for human beings to enjoy, and that pleasure is the only thing of ultimate or intrinsic worth are judgments of value. They don't tell us what it is right to do. For this we need a judgment of obligation. Under some ethical theories a judgment of obligation is dependent on, and follows directly from, a judgment of value. If an ethical theory does hold that judgments of obligation are dependent in this way, then it is what philosophers call a *teleological* or *consequentialist* theory of obligation. A teleological theory of obligation posits one and only one fundamental obligation and that is to maximize the good consequences and minimize the bad consequences of our actions. In so far as we need to know, under such theories, which consequences are good so that we can maximize them and which are bad so that we can minimize them, it is easy to see why a teleological theory of obligation presupposes a *theory of value*. Such a theory will provide us with the basis for justifying our judgments of value and thus ultimately our judgments of obligation.

The duty to maximize the good and minimize the bad consequences of our actions is the only fundamental duty under a teleological theory of obligation. On such a theory, then, any other obligations by which we feel bound, such as the obligation to honour our agreements or to tell the truth, are secondary and derivable from this one primary obligation. Mill's utilitarianism, as we shall see, is a teleological theory of obligation. In his view, all questions concerning what we ought to do are ultimately based on the principle of utility which requires that we maximize what is intrinsically good, namely, happiness or pleasure, and minimize what is intrinsically bad, unhappiness or pain. We have a duty to tell the truth, Mill would argue, but only because truth-telling is (normally) prescribed by the principle of utility.

In contrast to teleological theories of obligation there are those which are non-teleological. These we call *deontological theories* of obligation. Deontological theories of obligation essentially deny what teleological theories assert. They deny that we have one and only one fundamental duty, which is to maximize the good and minimize the bad consequences of our actions. There are basically two forms which this denial can take. First, a theory may suggest that the good and bad consequences of our actions have absolutely no bearing whatsoever on whether they are morally right or wrong. Such a strong deontological theory of obligation can operate wholly independently of any theory of value. We needn't know, as we do with teleological theories of obligation, what the good is if we are to know what we ought to do. The reason is simple: our obligation does not in any way involve the maximization of good consequences. Our duty is not to maximize what is ultimately of value and so we needn't have a theory of value which tells us what that is. Kant, as we shall see, appears to have held a strong deontological theory. Kant is notorious for suggesting that the rightness or wrongness of our actions is totally independent of whether or not they maximize good consequences. According to Kant, a judgment of obligation, like the judgment that health-care professionals must never withhold the truth from their patients, is in no way justified in terms of consequences. It is justified if and only if it meets the Categorical Imperative test which ignores consequences altogether.

A deontological theory of obligation need not, however, follow Kant's lead and claim that the consequences of our actions are completely irrelevant to their rightness or wrongness. There is a second kind of deontological theory which makes the weaker claim that good and bad consequences are not always the only things of moral importance. We have other ultimate obligations in addition to our duty to maximize the good and minimize the bad consequences of our actions. According to Ross, for example, the principle of beneficence, which requires promoting the good of others in our actions, is only one of many ultimate principles defining our moral obligations. Others include the obligation to be grateful for benefits given and the duty to be fair to other people. In Ross's view, we sometimes have a duty to be grateful even when neglecting this duty would on that occasion lead to the best consequences overall. Some actions, such as displays of gratitude are right, regardless of their consequences. Other actions, such as instances of unfairness, are sometimes wrong, even when they lead to good consequences.

Unlike Kant and Mill, then, Ross suggests that we have many fundamental obligations. The duty to be grateful and the duty to be fair are ultimate obligations which are not based on any more basic principle of obligation. This clearly separates Ross from Kant and Mill.

We frequently have a duty to be fair, Mill would urge, but this is because being fair normally maximizes the balance of good over bad consequences. Ross will have none of this. For him the duty to be fair is just as ultimate as the duty to maximize good consequences. We have many basic obligations and these cannot be reduced to any of the others. Ross's theory of obligation, insofar as it is not based on a single, fundamental principle defining a single, fundamental obligation is a *pluralist theory of obligation*. A pluralist theory of obligation, put simply, is one which does not posit a single, fundamental obligation upon which all other secondary obligations are based. A *monistic theory of obligation*, by contrast, does posit one such obligation. A utilitarian will be happy to talk of obligations to tell the truth or to be fair to others in our dealings with them. He will simply add that we have these obligations because fairness and truth-telling usually lead, in the end and all things considered, to the best consequences. Hence his theory is monistic. So too is Kant's.

To sum up, teleological theories of obligations are all logically dependent on theories of value. Some deontological theories of obligation are also dependent on a theory of value. Strong deontological theories such as Kant's exclude, as irrelevant, questions about the good or bad consequences of our actions (i.e. the value or disvalue to be realized in them). They therefore have no need of a theory of value. But most deontological theories do have such a need, since most deontological theories are pluralistic. Most are like Ross's in espousing principles which direct us, but not exclusively, to the good and bad consequences of our actions.

When we turn to theories of value, we find that these too may be categorized as either monistic or pluralistic. A *monistic theory of value*, as one might expect, posits one and only one thing, or characteristic of things, as being of value for its own sake. It posits, in other words, only one thing or characteristic as *intrinsically valuable*. Hedonism is one influential type of monistic theory of value. On this view, pleasure is the only thing which is valuable for its own sake. Anything else we value, say money or health, is valuable only *instrumentally*, as a means to the pleasure it brings. Classical utilitarianism, of the form espoused by Mill and his teacher Jeremy Bentham, is hedonistic. But it needn't be. Utilitarians who agree on a theory of obligation may divide on their theories of value. G.E. Moore, for instance, was a utilitarian like Mill. But unlike Mill, Moore espoused a *pluralistic theory of value* which saw pleasure as only one of many things of intrinsic value. Knowledge and aesthetic experience are among many other things worthy of pursuit for their own sakes.[2] If one holds a pluralistic theory of value, then one is faced with a difficulty: what to do in situations where two or more values conflict or cannot be pursued together. If freedom from manipulation and freedom from disease are both intrinsically valuable, then doctors may have to decide somehow between allowing their patients complete freedom of choice concerning their own medical treatment (thus risking bad decisions) and leading their patients to make what they, the doctors, think is the right choice. The question arises, however, whether it is possible to compare such very different values. Is comparing freedom from manipulation with freedom from disease, so as to see which is of greater value or importance in the circumstances, something that can be done rationally? Is an attempt to compare these two values a bit like trying to compare apples with oranges?

If, on the other hand, we adopt a monistic theory of value, we may seem to rid ourselves of such problems. We only have to compare, say, one pleasure with the next. But there are serious difficulties even here. How does one compare one person's pleasure with that of another, especially if those persons are as different as Bill Clinton and Pope John Paul II?

Monistic theories of value face another objection of some importance. According to many people there are numerous things in the world of ultimate, irreducible value. Friendship, for example, seems to be compromised if an attempt is made to reduce its value to the pleasure it brings. As will be seen, the attempt to place "value" on human lives and welfare is fraught with such difficulties. Some of these will be explored later in discussions concerning the propriety of utilizing "quality of life" as a criterion for decisions involving health care.

(6) Five Ethical Theories

Here follows a brief survey of five major types of ethical theory. The main reason for including the theories of Kant and Mill is that their contributions have dominated western moral thought since the scientific revolution. Kant strove to establish ethics as a purely rational enterprise while Mill believed that an objective standard of right and wrong could be discovered in the methods of the empirical sciences. If the rightness of our actions depends on the pleasure and pain they produce, then we ought to be able to estimate their rightness by empirical observation, measurements, and induction. Mill's utilitarianism is an ancestor of modern theories of cost-benefit analysis, which are assuming an ever-increasing role in controversies surrounding the allocation of money to various forms of health care.

Between them Kant and Mill zero in on the roles played respectively by intention and consequences in shaping our moral responses. One cannot get very far in discussions of ethics without paying deference to the Kantian notions of autonomy and universalizability, or the injunction to treat human beings as ends in themselves and not merely as means. Similarly one cannot ignore Mill's emphasis on protecting and promoting human happiness or well-being.

W.D. Ross's contribution to ethics is invaluable not only for its reaction to Kant and Mill, but because, in certain crucial respects, it seems more accurately to reflect the ordinary thinking and practice of moral agents than the more systematic reflections of professional moral philosophers. This is particularly evident in Ross's opposition to Kant's and Mill's reductionism in moral theory. Ross was unwilling to subscribe to a monistic theory of obligation. While acknowledging the powerful contributions of Kant and Mill to ethical theory, Ross resists elevating either the Categorical Imperative or the principle of utility to the status of a foundational first principle from which all other moral principles, rules, and judgments follow. In coming to grips with the moral issues considered in this text, it will be difficult to escape making reference to Ross's notion of *prima facie* duty.

Contemporary ethical theorists have experienced a renewed interest in the ethical writings of the ancient Greek philosopher, Aristotle. Among Aristotle's many contributions to the history of ethical thought is his doctrine of the mean. As we will see below, Aristotle attempts to isolate a number of virtues which we can more or less express or display in our lives when we aim for the *golden mean* between undesirable extremes. For example, we display the virtue courage when, in conducting our lives, we successfully steer clear of the extremes of cowardliness and foolhardiness. Courage is the mean between these two vices, and a courageous person is one whose character and (developed) dispositions lead him to act in neither a foolhardy nor a cowardly manner.

Those who are even more impressed than Ross with the immense complexity of moral life, and with the difficulties encountered when we try to articulate rules and principles to cover all cases, may find enormous potential in the Aristotelian approach. It is a consequence of Aristotle's conception of the moral life that there are no hard and fast rules or principles to tell us whether and to what extent our conduct approximates the relevant mean and is therefore virtuous. There are also no hard and fast rules to tell us what to do when our situation involves more than one virtue, as when our beneficence inclines us towards treating someone who would object were she informed about the matter, but our wish to be an honest person leads us in the other direction. In addressing moral questions we are not asking for rules which tell us what to do on some particular occasion. Rather, we are asking ourselves what kind of person we would be, what kinds of virtues we would display, were we to conduct our lives in a particular manner. And to these types of question there are almost never uniquely correct answers. Perhaps in this respect Aristotle's theory more accurately reflects our moral experience, and the humility of which we speak above in Section 4.

Finally, we have included a section on "feminist biomedical ethics." Feminist writings in biomedical ethics are characterized more by the approach taken to ethical theory than by any distinctive set of principles, rules, or values. Feminist bioethics is marked by a heightened concern for the personal and social *contexts* in which ethical decisions are made, and by the ways in which traditional ethical theory, with its attempt to discover universal, and therefore necessarily abstract, moral norms, ignores the context in which decisions are made. Of particular concern to feminists is the perceived failure of mainstream ethical theory to appreciate the context of oppressed individuals, like women and the socially vulnerable, and the various ways in which their legitimate concerns and interests are ignored, undervalued, or suppressed. In so far as medical practice has, until very recent times, been dominated by male physicians, and in so far as it involves, by its very nature, relationships with vulnerable individuals – patients – there is especially good reason to consider the lessons of feminist ethicists for biomedical practice.

(a) Utilitarianism

Utilitarianism is a monistic, teleological theory of obligation which, owing to its teleological nature, rests on a theory of value. A utilitarian's theory of value can of course be itself either monistic or pluralistic. We shall largely ignore the different theories of value espoused by utilitarians and concentrate instead on their theories of obligation.

Essentially there are two different kinds of utilitarianism, act and rule utilitarianism. Act utilitarianism (AU) defines the rightness or wrongness of individual actions in terms of the good or bad consequences realized by those actions themselves. In other words, AU defines the rightness or wrongness of an action in terms of its "utility" and "disutility." The term "utility" stands for whatever it is that is intrinsically valuable under the utilitarian's theory of value, "disutility" for whatever is thought to be intrinsically bad. According to John Stuart Mill, "actions are right in proportion as they tend to promote happiness; wrong as they tend to produce the reverse of happiness."[3] For him "utility" means happiness, and "disutility" unhappiness. Mill went on to identify happiness with pleasure and unhappiness with pain. Hence, Mill may be characterized as a *hedonistic* utilitarian, one on whose theory of value pleasure is the only thing of intrinsic worth. But a utilitarian need not make this identification, nor need he define utility in terms of happiness. Some utilitarians think it best to define utility in terms of the satisfaction of our actual preferences, while others would have us look to satisfy preferences we would have were we fully informed and rational. Regardless of the theory of value with which it is associated, however, AU always makes the following claim:

> AU: An act is right if and only if there is no other action I could have done instead which either (a) would have produced a greater balance of utility over disutility; or (b) would have produced a smaller balance of disutility over utility.

We must add (b) to account for those unfortunate situations where whatever we do we seem to cause more disutility than utility – where we're damned if we do and damned if we don't. In short, AU tells us to act always so as to bring about the best consequences we can, and sometimes that means trying to make the best of a bad situation.

AU was made famous in modern times by Mill and Bentham, at a time when it was quite natural for many people to think that some individuals simply count more than others. There were some who thought that members of the aristocracy, the Church, or a particular race were in some sense more worthy or superior than others and were therefore deserving of special consideration or privilege. The utilitarians were part of a social revolution which would have none of this. In the famous words of Bentham, "each is to count for one, none to count for more than one." In other words, according to utilitarians, *all* those affected by my actions should count *equally* in my deliberations concerning my moral obligations. The equal happiness of the King is to count equally with the equal happiness of the milk man. Mill put this important point in the following way:

> I must again repeat what the assailants of utilitarianism seldom have the justice to acknowledge, that the happiness which forms the utilitarian standard of what is right in conduct is *not* the agent's own happiness but that of all concerned. As between others, utilitarianism requires him to be as *strictly impartial as a disinterested benevolent spectator.*[4]

So built into AU is a commitment to equality and impartiality. We are to be concerned equally and impartially with the happiness or welfare, i.e. utility, of all those, including ourselves, who might be affected by our actions. On these grounds alone, AU is a very appealing theory. What could be better than to be sure that I always maximize, not my own happiness or that of my friends, but the happiness of all those people affected by my actions whoever they might be? What more could morality require?

Despite its inherently desirable features, many philosophers have come to find serious difficulties with AU. These have led some utilitarians to opt for an alternative form of the theory. One of the more serious difficulties for AU revolves around *special duties* and *special relationships*. These include duties of loyalty, of fidelity, and familial obligations. The latter rest in part on the special relationships which arise out of family ties and require some degree of partiality and special concern towards family members. It would be wrong, some think, to be impartial between friends and family, on the one hand, and perfect strangers on the other. It would be equally wrong to be impartial between one's patient and others who might benefit from the knowledge to be gained from using one's patient in an experiment. The importance of personal relationships in the moral evaluation of conduct is often stressed by feminists who reject the "impartiality" required by utilitarianism. In their view, treating everyone the same would be equivalent to treating them all as strangers.

Let us centre on promises to illustrate some of the most serious difficulties facing AU. Suppose I am a doctor and that a dear friend, Monica, comes to my clinic concerned that she might have AIDS. Monica has been unfaithful to her husband, Jack, whom I have also known for years. Our friendships go a long way back and are a continual source of happiness for all of us. Recent media discussions of the AIDS "epidemic" have got Monica worried. In order to ease her concern, I run the appropriate tests and determine that Monica has not been exposed to the HIV virus (the cause of AIDS). She is extremely relieved. Now she can continue her affair without worry. Her partner had a similar test done recently and so they are both clean. As Monica leaves my office she announces with a smile that of course she fully expects me to keep quiet about the test and the ongoing affair. Under no circumstances must Jack ever find out. She points out that as her physician I owe her a duty of confidentiality, a duty which is even stronger in this case, given our long friendship.

Upon reflection, however, I begin to wonder whether my duty does ultimately lie in confidentiality. I add up the utilities and disutilities involved for all affected by my decision, including not only Jack and Monica but their two young children and Monica's sexual partner. I correctly conclude that overall utility would be maximized, on balance, if I told Jack about the affair. He's a very reasonable and forgiving person and would likely be able to keep the marriage on the rails, something which would be of benefit to the entire family. As for Monica's partner, he will likely experience no difficulty in finding another sexual partner. As a consequence of my valid, act-utilitarian reasoning, I betray the confidence, despite my apparent duty as a physician and a friend. I consider it my moral obligation to maximize utility, even at the expense of harming a dear friend and violating a trust which has been placed in me.

Some philosophers believe that examples such as this show that AU takes promises, commitments, special relationships of trust, and so on, far too lightly. Indeed, some think it makes such factors totally irrelevant. This is because AU is a monistic theory of obligation which posits one and only one obligation – to maximize utility. Future consequences are all that count. Past commitments and special relationships are irrelevant.

A defender of AU, on the other hand, will likely reply that I have simply failed to consider all the relevant consequences. Of crucial importance here is not simply the fact that a marriage may be saved and a potentially destructive affair stopped, but also that my action will almost certainly destroy at least one valuable relationship (my friendship with Monica) which, in the long run, would add significantly to the utility I am able to bring about in my future actions. There is also the possibility that my betrayal will become common knowledge, thus threatening my role as a physician who can be trusted. Without my patients' trust, how can I practice medicine effectively? And if I cannot practice medicine effectively, how am I going to promote utility in my role as a doctor? Of course there's also the possibility that my action will weaken the public's trust of physicians in general – an even more disastrous possibility, viewed from the perspective of AU. All of these indirect consequences of breaking the agreement, when put into the balance, tip the scales in favour of keeping quiet. Those who think that AU takes special relationships and commitments far too lightly have simply ignored all the long-range, indirect effects of doing so.

So the defender of AU has a fairly forceful reply to such counter-examples to his theory of obligation. We should always be sure to ask, when a critic provides such an example: Have all the relevant consequences, long-range and indirect as well as immediate and direct, been accounted for? In all likelihood, they have not been. This is true whether we are talking about breaking confidences or violating autonomy.

Philosophers are fairly industrious when it comes to thinking up counter-examples to ethical theories. Having met replies such as the above, they have altered their counter examples to get rid of those convenient indirect, long-range effects upon which the defence is based. Some have dreamt up the *Desert Island Promise Case*, a version of which now follows.

You and a friend are alone on a deserted island. Your friend is dying and asks you to see to it when you are rescued that the elder of his two sons receives the huge sum of money your friend has secretly stashed away. You now are the only other person who knows of its existence. You solemnly promise to fulfil your friend's final request and he passes away secure in the knowledge that his last wish is in good hands. Upon rescue you are faced with a dilemma. The elder son turns out to be a lazy lout who squanders to no good end – even his own pleasure – whatever money he has. Even when he has lots of money to spend he still ends up being miserable and causing misery to other people. Your friend's younger son, however, is an aspiring researcher in dermatology. He is on the brink of uncovering a solution to the heartache of psoriasis, but will fail unless he receives financial backing. All his applications for grants have unjustly been denied and he has been left in desperation. As a good act utilitarian, you reason that utility would obviously be maximized if your solemn word to your dying friend were broken and you gave the money to the younger son. Think of all the utility that would be realized, all the suffering that would be alleviated! Compare this with the very little utility and considerable disutility that would result were you to give the money to the elder son.

Notice that in this case all the indirect, long-range consequences to which appeal was made in Monica's case are absent. No one will know that the promise is being broken and there are no valuable, utility-enhancing relationships in jeopardy. Your friend is dead. There seems little doubt in this situation that the promise should be broken according to AU – this is your moral obligation. But surely, the opponent will argue, this cannot be so. Solemn promises to dying friends, regardless of the good consequences which might be realized by breaking them, must be kept, except perhaps where disaster would result from keeping them. That it seems in such cases to give no weight at all to such promises shows that AU is a faulty theory of obligation. Solemn promises should weigh heavily – and independently of good consequences. Hence AU cannot be an adequate theory.

So promises and other such special commitments pose difficulties for AU. Free riders do too. Suppose there is a temporary but serious energy shortage in your community. All private homes and businesses have been requested to conserve electricity and gas. Private homes are to keep their thermostats no higher than 15 degrees centigrade and all businesses are temporarily to cut production by one-half. If everyone helps out in this way a serious overload which would prove disastrous will be avoided. Being a good act utilitarian, and knowing the tendencies of your neighbours, you reason as follows. "I know that everyone else will pay scrupulous attention to the government's request. So the potential disaster will be averted regardless of what I do. It will make no difference whatsoever if I run my production lines at two-thirds capacity. The little bit of extra electricity we use will have no negative effect at all. Of course if everyone ran at two-thirds, then disaster would result. But I know this is not going to happen and so the point is irrelevant. As for my employees, they will see a reduction and assume that the cut was to one-half, so no one will know but me.

Using two-thirds, then, will in no way prove harmful, but it will make a considerable amount of difference to my balance sheet. The extra production will enable the company to show a much higher profit this year. All things considered, then, it is morally permissible, indeed, my moral obligation, to run at two-thirds. This is what AU tells me that I should do."

Imagine the moral outrage which would result were your acting on this line of reasoning to become common knowledge. If the case seems far-fetched, consider how an analogous line of reasoning could be employed to justify extra diagnostic tests for your patient. Were you to pursue the recommended conduct, you would be labelled a "free rider," one who rides freely while others shoulder the burdens necessary for all to prosper. Your actions would be thought most unfair to all those who had willingly sacrificed their best interests, or the interests of their patients, for the good of everyone concerned. All this despite your efforts to maximize the utility of your actions.

In response to these (and similar) sorts of objections, some utilitarians have developed an alternative to AU. Consider further what would be said if your free riding came to light. The likely response would be to say: "Sure, no one is harmed if you use the extra electricity or prescribe the extra diagnostic tests. But imagine what would happen if everyone did what you are doing. Imagine if that became the norm. Disaster would result!" This request: "Imagine what would happen if everybody did that" has great probative force for many people. If *not everyone* could do what I propose to do without serious harm resulting, then many are prepared to say that it would be wrong for *anyone* to do it, and hence wrong for me to do it. In response to the force of this intuition, some utilitarians have developed a very different variety of their theory called *rule utilitarianism* (RU). On this version the rightness or wrongness of an action is not to be judged by its consequences. Rather it is to be judged by the consequences of everyone's adopting a *general rule* under which the action falls.

As an introduction to RU, consider a case outlined by John Rawls in his famous paper "Two Concepts of Rules."[5] Rawls has us imagine that we are a sheriff in the deep American south. The rape of a white woman has taken place and although the identity of the rapist is unknown, it is clear that the offender was black. The predominantly white and racially bigoted community is extremely agitated over the incident and great social unrest is threatening. Riots are about to break out and many innocent, and possibly some not so innocent, people will be killed. If you were able to identify and arrest the rapist, the unrest would undoubtedly subside; but unfortunately you have no leads, other than the fact that the rapist was black. It occurs to you that you do not really need the actual culprit to calm things down. Why not simply concoct a case against a randomly chosen black man who has no alibi and have him arrested? The crowd will be placated, and although one innocent man will suffer, many innocent lives will be saved.

Rawls uses this example to illustrate an apparent weakness in AU and how RU allows one to overcome it. The consequences of framing the (possibly) innocent black are far better (or less bad), in terms of utility, than allowing the riot to occur. Hence AU seems to require the frame, a course of action which is clearly unjust. Of course the defender of AU has several tricks up his sleeve at this point. He can once again appeal to the possible indirect effects of the frame. Suppose the lie came to light. Terrible social paranoia and unrest would result; people would no longer trust the judicial system and would wonder constantly whether they might be next. Indirect consequences such as these, the defender of AU will argue, clearly outweigh any short-term, direct benefits. But Rawls suggests that we consider a different question than the one AU would have us ask. We are to consider whether a general rule which permits the framing of innocent persons could possibly figure in a moral code general acceptance of which would result in the maximization of utility. If it could not (which is surely the case), then the proposed frame is morally impermissible. Since no such general rule could find its way into an acceptable moral code, largely for the reasons mentioned above in the parenthetical aside, an action in accordance with that rule would be morally wrong. Hence it would be morally wrong on RU to frame the possibly innocent black, even if the consequences of that particular action would be better than those of the alternatives. We are not morally required, on RU, to perform actions which individually would maximize utility. Rather we are to perform actions which accord with a set of rules whose general observance would maximize utility. Actions are judged according to whether they conform with acceptable rules; only the rules themselves are judged in terms of utility. The essence of RU is expressed in the following claim:

RU: An act is morally right if and only if it conforms with a set of rules whose general observance would maximize utility.

One extremely important difference between RU and AU is worth stressing. It is quite possible, on RU, to be required to perform an action which does not, on that particular occasion, maximize utility. Observance of the best set of general rules does not, on each individual occasion, always lead to the best consequences. Of course it *generally* does, but there are exceptions. This is something the defender of RU seems willing to live with for the sake of overall, long-term utility gains and the ability to deal with desert-island promises, free riders, and so on.

RU is not without its difficulties, however. Some utilitarians claim, for example, that RU really does violate the spirit of utilitarianism and amounts to "rule worship."[6] If the ideal behind utilitarianism is the maximization of utility, then should we not be able to deviate from the generally acceptable rules when doing so will serve to maximize utility? If the defender of RU allows exceptions to be made in such cases, then he runs the risk of collapsing his RU into AU. The rules would no longer hold any special weight or authority in our moral decisions. We would end up following the rules when it is best to do so and depart from them when that seems best.[7] In each case we seem led to do what AU requires, namely, maximize the utility of our individual actions. If, on the other hand, the defender of RU holds fast and says we must *never* deviate from rules which generally advance utility but sometimes do not, then the charge of rule worship comes back to plague the utilitarian.

A second problem facing RU can be summed up in an example. Suppose it were true that the best set of rules for the circumstances of our society would place an obligation on first-born children to provide for their elderly parents. I, the younger of two sons, reason that I therefore have no obligation whatsoever to provide for my elderly parents, even though I know that my elder brother is unwilling to provide more than the 50 per cent he thinks we each ought to provide. My parents end up living a life of abject poverty on only 50 per cent of what they need to sustain themselves. Something seems clearly wrong here. Our obligations, it would seem, cannot be entirely a function of an *ideal code* which may never in fact be followed by anyone except me. We seem to require, in an acceptable moral theory, some recognition of how other people are behaving, what rules they are in fact following. The rules they are following may be perfectly acceptable but not ideal, in which case I should perhaps follow them too. This is as true in medicine as it is elsewhere. Serious harm might result were an idealistic physician to act according to an ideal code, general observance of which would maximize utility, when no one else was prepared to do so. Perhaps here the excuse, "But no one else is willing to do it" carries some weight.

To sum up, there are significant differences between AU and RU and neither theory is free from difficulty. AU requires that we always seek, on each particular occasion, to maximize utility. It has difficulties with, among other things, free riders, desert-island promises, and sheriffs tempted by good consequences to commit injustice. RU tells us to perform actions which conform to a set of rules general observance of which would lead to the best consequences overall. This theory seems to provide solutions to many of the problems plaguing AU but it does so only at the expense of introducing new puzzles of its own. It must somehow provide a bridge between the best ideal code and the actual beliefs, practices, and accepted rules of one's society, all the while steering a course between rule worship and a straightforward reduction to AU.

(b) Deontological Ethics – Immanuel Kant

Kant, like Mill, proposes a monistic theory of obligation. Unlike, Mill, however, the theory is thoroughly non-consequentialist. It denies that the possible consequences of our actions are what determine their rightness or wrongness. According to Kant,

> An action done from duty has its moral worth, not in *the purpose* [i.e. the consequences] to be attained by it, but in the maxim in accordance with which it is decided upon; it depends, therefore, not on the realization of the object of the action, but solely on the *principle of volition* [the maxim] in accordance with which, irrespective of all objects of the faculty of desire [i.e. pleasure, happiness, preferences] the action has been performed.[8]

In this remark we see clearly that Kant espouses a deontological theory of obligation. The morality of an action is determined not by its consequences but by the maxim, the general principle, to which it conforms. Its moral worth lies not in the happiness or pleasure it produces, but in the kind of action it is. Let's try to clarify this point.

A key notion in Kant's theory is the notion of a maxim. By this technical term Kant means a general rule or principle which specifies what it is I conceive myself as doing and my reason for doing it. For example, suppose I decide to tell a lie in order to avoid distress to my patient. The maxim of my action could be expressed in the following way: "Whenever I am able to avoid distress to my patient by lying, I shall do so." This maxim makes plain that I conceive myself as lying and that my reason is the avoidance of a patient's distress. It makes plain that I consider the avoidance of such distress as a *sufficient reason* to lie. Were I to act on my maxim I would in effect be expressing my commitment to a general rule which extends in its scope beyond the particular situation in which I find myself. In supposing that the avoidance of patient distress is a sufficient reason in that situation to lie, I commit myself to holding that in any other situation just like it, i.e. any other case in which a lie would serve to avoid a patient's distress, I should tell a lie. This *generalizability of reasons* and maxims can perhaps be illustrated through an example involving a non-moral judgment.

Suppose you and I are baseball fans.

I say to you, "The Toronto Blue Jays are a good baseball team because their team batting average is about .260 and the average ERA among their starting pitchers is under 3.50."

You reply, "What is your opinion of the Montreal Expos?"

I say, "They are a lousy team."

You reply, "But their team batting average is also about .260 and the average ERA among their starters is 3.4."

I am stuck here in a logical inconsistency. I must either modify my earlier assessment of the Blue Jays – say that they too are a lousy team – or admit that the Expos are also a good team. By citing my reasons for judging the Blue Jays a good ball team, I commit myself to a general maxim that *any* baseball team with a team batting average of over .260 and whose starting rotation has an ERA of below 3.50 is a good baseball team. If I don't agree with the implications of that general maxim, e.g. I still think the Expos are a bad ball team, then logical consistency demands that I reject or modify the maxim. Perhaps I will add that in addition to a team batting average of over .260 and a ERA among starting pitchers of under 3.5, a good baseball team must have several "clutch" players. I would add this if I thought that the absence of clutch players explains why the Expos, unlike the Blue

Jays, are not a good team. Of course I could make this alteration only if I thought the Blue Jays did have at least a few clutch players.

So my maxim that whenever I can avoid distress to my patient by lying I shall do so, insofar as it expresses a general reason, applies to other situations similar to the one in which I initially act upon it. But this is not the full extent of my commitment. If avoiding patient distress really is a sufficient reason for *my* telling a lie, then it must also be a sufficient reason for *anyone else* who finds herself in a situation just like mine. According to Kant, and virtually all moral philosophers, acting upon a maxim commits me, as a rational moral agent, to a *universal* moral rule governing all persons in situations just like mine (in the relevant respects). I must be prepared to accept that a sufficient reason for me is a sufficient reason for anyone else in precisely my situation. This is the force of the first formulation of Kant's Categorical Imperative we are about to consider. If I think some other person in a position to avoid patient distress by lying should not tell the lie, then I must either retract my earlier maxim or specify some relevant difference between our situations, as I did when I tried to show that the Expos are a bad baseball team despite their strong team batting average and pitching staff.

Acting for reasons, that is, acting rationally (which is required, according to Kant if we are to be moral), commits me to universal rules or maxims which I must be prepared to accept. Kant expresses this point in terms of my capacity to will that my personal maxim should become a *universal law*. According to the first formulation of the Categorical Imperative, the fundamental principle of obligation in Kant's monistic system, "I ought never to act except in such a way that *I can also will that my maxim should become a universal law.*"[9] Later he writes, "*Act as if the maxim of your action were to become through your will a universal law of nature.*"[10] According to Kant, immoral maxims and the immoral actions based upon them can never, under any conceivable circumstances, pass the Categorical Imperative test. This is not, as we shall now see, because the consequences of general observance of an immoral maxim would be undesirable in terms of utility. Rather it is because the state of affairs in which the maxim is observed as a universal law is *logically impossible* or *inconceivable* – it involves us in contradiction.

Some states of affairs simply cannot exist, in the strongest sense of "cannot." The state of affairs in which I am, at one and the same time, Rob's father *and* Rob's son is logically impossible. It cannot exist. Were I for some strange reason to will that this state of affairs exist, my will, Kant would say, would contradict itself. It would be willing inconsistent, contradictory things: that I am Rob's father and son at one and the same time. Now consider a case actually discussed by Kant. Suppose that a man

> finds himself driven to borrowing money because of need. He well knows that he will not be able to pay it back; but he sees too that he will get no loan unless he gives a firm promise to pay it back within a fixed time. He is inclined to make such a promise; but he has still enough conscience to ask "Is it not unlawful and contrary to duty to get out of difficulties in this way?" Supposing, however, he did resolve to do so, the maxim of his action would run thus, "Whenever I believe myself short of money, I will borrow money and promise to pay it back, though I know that this will never be done." Now this principle of self-love or personal advantage is perhaps quite compatible with my own entire future welfare; only there remains the question "Is it right?" I therefore transform the demand of self love into a universal law and frame my question thus, "How would things stand if my maxim became a universal law?" I then see straight away that this maxim can never rank as a universal law of nature and be self-consistent, but must necessarily contradict itself. For the universality of a law that every one believing himself to be in need can make any promise he pleases with the intention not to keep it would make promising, and the very purpose of promising, itself impossible, since no one would believe he was being promised anything, but would laugh at utterances of this kind as empty shams.[11]

It is important to be clear exactly what Kant is saying in this passage. He is not objecting to insincere promises on the ground that they will cause others to lose confidence in us and mean that we will jeopardize the valuable consequences of future promises. Nor is he arguing that false promises contribute to a general mistrust of promises and the eventual collapse of a valuable social practice. These are all *consequentialist* considerations which, according to the deontologist Kant, are totally irrelevant to questions of moral obligation. His point is a very different one. He is suggesting that a state of affairs in which everyone in need makes false promises is incoherent. There is a *contradiction* because, on the one hand, everyone in need *would* borrow on false promises. They would be following the maxim "as a law of nature," with the same regularity as the planets observe Kepler's laws of planetary motion. Yet on the other hand, in this very same state of affairs no one *could* borrow on a false promise, because if such promises were always insincere, no one would be stupid enough to lend any money. Promising requires trust on the part of the promisee, but in the state of affairs contemplated there just couldn't be any, and so promises of the sort in question would simply be impossible. Hence any attempt to will, as a universal law of nature, the maxim "Whenever I believe myself short of money, I will borrow money and promise to pay it back, though I know that this will never be done," lands us in contradiction. "I... see straight away that this maxim can never rank as a universal law of nature and be self-consistent, but must necessarily contradict itself."[12]

With Kant, then, we have a moral test of our actions which does not lie in an assessment of their consequences. Nor does the test lie in weighing the consequences of adopting a general rule which licences those actions. Rather the test considers the logical coherence of the universalized maxim upon which I personally propose to act. Whether this test successfully accounts for all of our moral obligations is highly questionable. Is there anything incoherent in the state of affairs in which everyone kills his neighbour if she persists in playing her stereo at ear-piercing levels? Such a state of affairs might be highly *undesirable* (though some days I really do wonder) but it seems perfectly possible or conceivable. Yet killing off annoying neighbours seems hardly the right thing to do.

Kant provided two further formulations of his Categorical Imperative. He thought these versions equivalent to the first, though it is difficult to see why Kant thought this to be so. The equivalence question needn't concern us here however. The additional formulations bring to light two important principles which many people find highly appealing and which may prove helpful in dealing with some of the problems discussed later in this text.

According to Kant, if I act only on maxims which could, without contradiction, serve as universal laws I will never treat people as *mere means to my ends*. The Categorical Imperative requires that I "Act in such a way that [I] always treat humanity, whether in [my] own person or in the person of any other, never simply as a means, but always at the same time as an end."[13] In more common terms, we should never just *use* people. The emphasis here is on the *intrinsic worth* and *dignity* of rational creatures. I treat rational beings as ends in themselves if I respect in them the same value I discover in myself, namely, my freedom to determine myself to action and to act for reasons which I judge for myself. As Kant observes, there can be nothing more dreadful to a rational creature than that his actions should be subject to the will of another. I treat others as mere things rather than as persons, subject them to my will in the way I do a tool, if I fail to respect their dignity. This principle has an important role to play in assessing, for example, the doctor-patient relationship, the requirement of informed, valid consent to medical experimentation, and requests for physician-assisted suicide.

Kant's third formulation of the Categorical Imperative seems closely tied to the second. In effect, it spells out what it is in rational agents which gives them their dignity and worth. It requires that we treat others as *autonomous* agents, capable of self-directed, rational action. The capacity to rise above the compelling forces of desire, self-interest, and physical necessity, to act freely on the basis of *reasons*, is what gives rational beings their dignity and worth. To treat a person as an end in herself, then, is to respect her autonomy and freedom. As noted, it rules out various kinds of manipulative practices and paternalistically motivated behaviours. In a case involving asbestos poisoning at Johns Manville,[14] company doctors neglected to tell workers the alarming results of their medical tests. This was rationalized on the ground that there was nothing that could be done to curb the disease anyway, and so the workers were better off not knowing. Such paternalistic conduct clearly violated Kant's Categorical Imperative. It failed to respect the autonomy and dignity of the asbestos workers. Of course the conduct might have been fully justified by AU, though this point is open to argument. Whether in the long run such deceptions serve to maximize utility is perhaps questionable.

With Kant we have a clear alternative to the monistic, teleological theory of obligation provided by the act and rule utilitarians. Kant's theory is clearly deontological and is at the very least monistic in its intent. Kant attempts to ground all our obligations on one fundamental principle: the Categorical Imperative. As we have seen, Kant provides three formulations of this principle, though it is difficult to see how they are exactly equivalent. In any event, we may view Kant as requiring that we ask the following three questions:

1. Could I consistently will, as a universal law, the personal maxim upon which I propose to act?
2. Would my action degrade other rational agents or myself by treating them or myself as a mere means?
3. Would my action violate the autonomy of some rational agent, possibly myself?

Should any of these three questions yield the wrong answer, my moral obligation is to refrain from acting on my personal maxim.

(c) Ethical Pluralism – W.D. Ross

Ross's theory of obligation arose mainly out of his dissatisfaction with utilitarian theories. While Ross's main target was G.E. Moore, his criticisms are relevant to utilitarianism in general, particularly AU. According to Ross, utilitarianism in all of its guises grossly oversimplifies the moral relationships between people. As we have seen, utilitarianism is, in the end, concerned solely with the maximization of utility. Our concern should rest exclusively with the overall consequences of our actions, or the rules under which we perform them. In Ross's view, morality should acknowledge the importance of consequences, but not exclusively. Utilitarianism errs in thinking that consequences are all that matter, in thinking that "the only morally significant relationship in which my neighbours stand to me is that of being possible beneficiaries [or victims] of my action."[15] It errs, in other words, in being a monistic, teleological theory of obligation. Ross proposes instead a pluralistic theory of obligation which recognizes several, irreducible moral relationships and principles. In addition to their role as possible beneficiaries of my actions, my fellow human beings "may also stand to me in the relation of promisee to promiser, of creditor to debtor, of wife to husband, of child to parent, of friend to friend, of fellow countryman to fellow countryman, and the like."[16] "The like" no doubt includes the relation of doctor to patient, doctor to nurse, experimenter to subject and so on, relationships which are integral to the health-care professions and which are ignored only at the cost of moral confusion.

In Ross's view, utilitarianism not only oversimplifies the moral relationships in which we stand to others, it also distorts the whole basis of morality by being thoroughly teleological in orientation. On utilitarian theories we must always be *forward-looking* to the future consequences of our actions or rules. But sometimes, Ross urges, morality requires that we look *backwards* to what has occurred in the past. There is significance, for example, in the sheer fact that a promise has been made, a promise which has moral force independent of any future good consequences that might arise from keeping it. This moral force explains why we should normally keep promises made to dying friends even if utility would be maximized were we to break them. A promise itself, because of the *kind* of action it is, has a moral force which is totally independent of its consequences. Teleological theories, because they ignore such features and are entirely forward-looking, distort morality. *Promises, contracts, commitments* to serve a certain role, *agreements, loyalty, friendship* and so on, all have moral force, and all can give rise to obligations and responsibilities independently of good or bad consequences.

Ross provides us, then, with a pluralistic, deontological theory of obligation. In this theory we find a plurality of ultimate principles, only some of which are consequentialist in orientation. According to Ross, each of these principles specifies a *prima facie* duty or obligation. These are duties which we must fulfil *unless* we are also, in the circumstances, subject to another, competing prima facie duty of greater weight. We have a prima facie duty to tell the truth, which means that we must always tell the truth unless a more stringent duty applies to us and requires a falsehood. An example from Kant helps to illustrate this feature nicely.

Kant is notorious for arguing that the Categorical Imperative establishes an unconditional duty always to tell the truth. He has us consider a case where a murderer comes to our door asking for the whereabouts of his intended victim. Should we tell him the truth, that the victim is seeking refuge in our house, and thereby become accomplices in his murder? Both AU and RU would undoubtedly licence a lie under such extraordinary circumstances, but according to Kant the Categorical Imperative does not. The duty to tell the truth is unconditional, despite the consequences of its observance. "To be truthful (honest) in all declarations... is a sacred and absolutely commanding decree of reason, limited by no expediency."[17] According to Ross's theory this is not so. Kant's case is clearly one where our prima facie duty to be truthful is overridden or outweighed by more stringent duties to our friend.

Ross's list of prima facie duties provides a helpful classification of some of the various duties and morally significant relationships recognized in our everyday moral thinking. There are:

1. Duties resting on previous actions of our own. These include:
   (a) duties of *fidelity* arising from explicit or implicit promises;
   (b) duties of *reparation*, resting on previous wrongful acts of ours and requiring that we compensate, as best we can, the victims of our wrongful conduct.
2. Duties resting on the services of others; duties of *gratitude* which require that we return favour for favour.
3. Duties involving the *fair* distribution of goods; duties of *justice*, which require fair sharing of goods to be distributed.
4. Duties to improve the condition of others; duties of *beneficence* (which in part form the basis of utilitarian theories of obligation).
5. Duties to improve our own condition; duties of *self-improvement*.
6. Duties not to injure others; duties of *non-maleficence*.[18]

Ross's list of duties is by no means exhaustive, and no doubt many would quarrel with some of the duties Ross has included. For instance, it might be questioned whether duties of self-improvement belong on a list of *moral* duties. It is plausible to suppose that moral duties arise only in our relationships with other people; that the demands of morality govern inter-personal relationships only. Allowing one's talents to lie unused or allowing one's health to deteriorate may be imprudent or foolish, but is it immoral? Perhaps it is if others, say our children, are depending on us. But in this case it's not a moral duty of self-improvement which is violated but rather duties such as the duties of beneficence and possibly non-maleficence. Another questionable candidate is the duty to be grateful. If someone does me a favour, is it true that I am required, as a matter of duty, to be grateful? Is gratitude something that can be subject to duty, or is it rather something that must be freely given, given not out of a sense of duty but out of genuine, heartfelt goodwill? If a favour is done with the sense that something is *owing* as a result, then perhaps it is not really a favour at all, but an investment.

In any case, the intention here is not to take issue with Ross's list – only to suggest that specific items are perhaps open to question. This leads to a point of some significance. According to Ross, that we have the prima facie duties he mentions is simply *self-evident* to any rational human being who thinks seriously about the requirements of morality. The existence of these duties, and the validity of the principles which describe them, are known through *moral intuition*. To say that a principle is self-evident and known through intuition is to say that its truth is evident to an attentive mind, that it neither needs supporting evidence nor needs to be deduced from other propositions. It stands alone as something obviously true. In this instance, it stands alone as something whose truth is known directly through *moral* intuition.

This feature of Ross's theory is very controversial among philosophers, who are generally suspicious of "self-evident principles" and "intuition." In the case of morality, the apparent obviousness of some principles, and the certainty with which many believe them, seem better explained by such things as uniform moral upbringing and common experiences. And then there is the problem of disagreement. If a principle truly is self-evident, then should not everyone agree on its validity? Yet this is seldom, if ever, the case with moral principles, including those on Ross's list.

This is not the place to discuss further the reasons behind the philosopher's suspicions concerning self-evidence and moral intuition, except to add the following. One who claims self-evidence for his views has little to say to those holding conflicting self-evident claims. He can ask that we think again, but he cannot undertake to prove his claims to us. If his claims truly are self-evident and known through intuition, they are in need of no proof. Perhaps more importantly, none can be given. So if, after careful reflection, you continue to disagree with some of the principles on Ross's list, he has little recourse but to accuse you of moral blindness. He must view you as equivalent to a person who cannot see the difference between red and blue; your moral blindness is on a par with his colour blindness. One might ask whether this is a satisfactory response to serious moral disagreements among reasonable people of good will and integrity.

Ross believes that his self-evident principles articulate prima facie moral obligations. These are obligations which hold unless overridden in individual cases by a more stringent or weightier duty. As for how we are to determine which of two or more prima facie duties has greater weight in a given case, Ross provides no answer except to say that we must use our best judgment. This is of little help because it fails to tell us the considerations upon which our judgments are to be based. Ross is fully aware that in most cases of conflicting obligations it is far from clear which duty is more stringent. Reasonable people of moral integrity will disagree. We therefore seem left with a serious gap in the theory and must either accept that in cases of conflict there is no one right thing to do, that the best we can do is fulfil one of our conflicting duties and violate the other; or we must continue to look for a *criterion* in terms of which conflicts can be resolved.

It is at this point that the utilitarian will be more than happy to offer assistance. In his view, Ross has isolated the basis for a set of rules which are indeed important in everyday moral thinking. According to the defender of AU, these Rossian rules are useful guidelines or rules of thumb which we are well advised in most cases to follow. If we follow them regularly, our actions will in the long run end up maximizing utility. The act of promising usually does maximize utility, as does a display of gratitude. But in those cases in which a conflict in the rules arises, or where an applicable rule seems inappropriate for good utilitarian reasons, we must resort directly to the AU criterion and decide which action will maximize utility. As for the proponent of RU, he will likely claim that Ross's rules will almost certainly figure in the set of rules general observance of which within a modern society will maximize utility. He too is likely to claim that in cases in which the rules conflict direct recourse must be made to the principle of utility. We must follow the rule which in the circumstances will lead to the maximization of utility. Of course Ross must reject the utilitarian's offer of rescue. Were he to follow the utilitarian's lead he would in effect be adopting the principle of utility as defining a single, ultimate obligation, and this would be to deny Ross's central claim that each of his prima facie duties is ultimate and irreducible. But then it is far from clear how this plurality of irreducible duties is to be dealt with in cases of conflict. We seem truly left with a serious gap. Without a means of adjudicating among conflicting prima facie duties, we are left short just where we need guidance the most.

(d) Virtue Ethics – Aristotle
(i) What should we be? versus What ought we to do?
Despite their many differences, the theories of Kant, Ross, and the utilitarians had at least one thing in common: they were all designed to answer directly the question "What ought I to do?" In other words, these theories were designed to help us determine what action(s) we should perform in particular circumstances. The concern, in short, was with the rightness of actions, with determining wherein our duty lies. According to Kant, the question "What ought I to do?" is

answered by determining whether the maxim of one's action can be universalized. For rule utilitarians the answer lies in whether the rule(s) under which one acts maximize(s) overall utility. Although act utilitarians believe that rules have no role in our moral reasoning, except as rules of thumb, the question remains: "What is the right thing for me to do in these circumstances?" According to act utilitarians, we answer this question by determining which of the actions open to us would maximize utility. Ross too was concerned to help us determine what we should do in particular circumstances, with determining the course of (right) action wherein our moral duty lies. Modern theories sometimes transform the questions of Mill, Ross, and Kant into questions about our rights, but still the emphasis is on the evaluation of actions, on determining what we have a right to do.

Much earlier in the history of moral philosophy, the Greek philosopher Aristotle sought to cast ethics in an entirely different mould. This is a mould which some contemporary moral philosophers find highly appealing partly because it allows us to avoid many of the difficulties encountered by the traditional deontological and utilitarian theories, but also because it is thought to provide a much better understanding of our moral lives, what it is we strive to be in pursuing the moral life and why the moral life is important to us. The fundamental ethical question for Aristotle is not "What ought I to *do*?" but "What should I *be*?" As one similarly minded theorist put it,

> ... morality is internal. The moral law ... has to be expressed in the form, "be this," not in the form "do this." ... the true moral law says "hate not," instead of "kill not." ... the only mode of stating the moral law must be as a rule of character.[19]

For Aristotle, moral behaviour expresses *virtues* or qualities of *character*. There is a much greater emphasis on "character traits" and "types of persons," than on rules, obligations, duties, and rights. Aristotle is interested in questions such as these: Should we *be* niggardly or generous? Hateful or benevolent? Cowardly or courageous? Over-indulgent or temperate? In what do these traits consist? How are they cultivated? And how do they figure in a life well lived? In discussing these questions about the character traits integral to moral life, Aristotle offered exemplars of virtue to emulate and vices to avoid rather than rules or principles to be obeyed or disobeyed. In short, for Aristotle, morality is *character oriented* rather than *rule driven.* Aristotle would no doubt have frowned on modern ethical theories which divorce actions and questions about them from the character of moral (or immoral) agents who perform them. Aristotle was not interested in the mere doing of actions, but also with the character of the doer from whom actions flow. Praiseworthy and blameworthy actions are not those which match up to a particular template of rules or principles, but rather ones which flow from and reveal a certain type of character. Moral agency is not merely a matter of which rules to follow, but a whole way of life which requires a unity of thought and feeling which is characteristic of what Aristotle called "virtue."

(ii) Theoretical and Practical Reason

Aristotle divided knowledge into the theoretical and the practical. *Episteme* is concerned with speculative or theoretical inquiries, and its object is knowledge of the truth. This was contrasted with *phronesis* or practical knowledge which focuses on what is "*doable*" rather than on what is *knowable* for its own sake. Without *phronesis*, particular virtues of character (e.g., courage, moderation, and generosity) would not be achievable by human beings, and the conduct which flows from and expresses these virtues would not be likely. It is central to Aristotle's view of human knowledge and moral excellence that whereas the intellectual virtues associated with *episteme* can be acquired through teaching, the virtues of character achievable via phronesis require practice until they become "second nature." Moral virtue can not just be taught, it requires "training" and "habituation," the doing of virtuous actions. In order to be a virtuous person one must develop the disposition to be virtuous; and this requires training and the doing of virtuous actions till this becomes a settled disposition.

(iii) Human Good

Aristotle's ethical theory is teleological. "Every art and every inquiry, every action and choice, seems to aim at some good; whence the good has rightly been defined as that at which all things aim."[20] There are different goods corresponding to the various arts and modes of inquiry. Seamanship aims at safe voyages, the musical arts at the creation of beautiful music, and the medical arts aim at health. Is there, Aristotle asks, a good for human beings as such? If so, then perhaps we can begin to understand what we might call the art of living well by considering what is necessary to the achievement of that end? Just as we can understand proper medical practice in relation to the good which medicine strives to achieve, perhaps we can also understand moral life in relation to the good for humans which moral life strives to achieve. So Aristotle is interested in action in so far as it contributes to the good for human beings. The right thing to do is best understood in relation to what is conducive to the good for human beings, just as a "proper prescription" is best understood in relation to what is conducive to the patient's health.

In his classic work, the *Nicomachean Ethics*, Aristotle confines his discussion of the good, that at which all things aim, to human good. The good aimed at by human beings is *eudaemonia*, usually translated as "happiness" or "well-being."[21] Some people identify human good with such things as wealth, pleasure, and honour, but Aristotle quickly shows that these people cannot be right. Wealth, for example, is at best a (very unreliable) means to happiness, not happiness itself. Pleasure is not the good for human beings even though it is true, as Aristotle's teacher Plato argued, that the good person takes pleasure in virtuous activity. Pleasure is not itself the good, but only an external sign of the presence of goodness. One will experience pleasure when one does things well; doing well does not consist in the achievement of pleasure. In Aristotle's sense of the term, happiness or well-being is something enjoyed over a lifetime in the exercise of virtues such as courage, moderation, and generosity of spirit. In one sense the exercise of the virtues is a means to the achievement of happiness or well-being. In a deeper sense it is not. The exercise of virtue is integral to the achievement of happiness, constitutive of it, not merely a prepayment of dues to insure happiness. In short, the virtuous life is not a means to the end of well-being; it *is* the life of well-being.

(iv) Virtue

Central to the Aristotelian conception of ethics and the good life is, as we have seen, the notion of "virtue." Aristotle's definition of this key notion is as follows. Virtue is "a state of character concerned with choice, lying in a mean, i.e. the mean relative to us, this being determined by rational principle, that principle by which the man of practical wisdom would determine it..."[22] The key notions in this definition need to be clarified.

A central element in Aristotle's conception of virtue is "disposition." Virtue, as we will see, is a kind of disposition. William

Frankena summarizes the nature of dispositions as follows:

> ... dispositions or traits ... are not wholly innate; they must all be acquired, at least in part, by teaching and practice, or, perhaps by grace. They are also traits of "character," rather than traits of "personality" like charm or shyness, and they all involve a tendency to do certain kinds of action in certain kinds of situations, not just to think or feel in certain ways. They are not just abilities or skills, like intelligence or carpentry, which one may have without using.[23]

Linguistically, terms describing dispositions are often contrasted with "occurrence" terms. A dispositional term like "timid" tells us a good deal more about a person than the occurrence word "frightened." The former tells us something about the character of the individual whereas the latter may tell us nothing more than that the person was in a particular state on some occasion or other. It is possible that the state we might call "Tom's being frightened" occurred on some occasion even though Tom has no disposition to be frightened. Very little future behaviour can be predicted from being told that someone is frightened or angry, even if we know the reasons why he is frightened or angry. On the other hand, if we are told that Jack is timid or irascible, then we can predict that he will tend to get frightened or angry in circumstances that would not frighten or anger other people with a more courageous or gentler disposition. Having such dispositions does not, of course, rule out the possibility of sometimes acting "out of character." There are provocations that would try even the patience of Job, some tasks so dangerous as to deter the most courageous and resolute persons, and some offers that even the most conscientious person cannot refuse. Dispositions, as tendencies, have an elasticity about them.

Aristotle's definition of virtue begins with virtue as a disposition, but it does not end there. Virtue is a disposition *to choose well*. Commenting on the etymology of the Greek word for choice, *prohairesis*, Aristotle writes: "the very term *prohairesis* ... denotes something chosen before other things."[24] Choosing something before other things requires (a) the presence of alternatives. Without alternatives there can be no choice. It also requires (b) deliberation about the relative merits of the alternatives open to the agent. Virtuous actions are principled and thoughtful. They are responses rather than reactions.

Deliberation about the alternatives open to the agent requires (c) ranking of those alternatives. One alternative is preferred to another and chosen. Finally, *prohairesis* presupposes (d) voluntarism. Virtue requires that we are responsible for our own actions. We are the begetters or efficient causes of our own actions, agents not patients. Our actions must be "self-caused," i.e., "in our power and voluntary."[25]

Aristotle emphasizes that primarily choice is restricted to means and not ends. The ultimate and remote end of our choosing, *eudaemonia* or happiness, is fixed by human nature. Just as all things within the universe have an essential nature (understood by Aristotle in terms of a unique function the thing serves) in relation to which their "good" can be understood, human nature provides a natural basis for understanding the good for human beings. This particular feature of Aristotle's view allows him to avoid arbitrariness in his ethics; ethics is not based on variable social norms or customs, or on the personal predilections of individuals or groups of individuals. Ethics is not "culturally relative" or "subjective" on this account; it is grounded in nature and to that extent "objective." Although the "objectivity" of the Aristotelian schema allows Aristotle to avoid relativism, it is a serious source of concern for some. Many critics see danger in the idea that there is a largely fixed, essential human nature in terms of which the moral life, and the requirements it places upon us, are to be understood. Some followers of Aristotle have argued that procreation is "natural" to human beings (as it is to all organisms) and that so-called "artificial" means of reproduction are therefore inherently suspicious and perhaps even immoral. Others take a similar line of argument in supporting the view that homosexuality is immoral. Whether such views follow from the Aristotelian system, and whether Aristotle would himself accept the views attributed to his conception, are highly questionable. But there is, nevertheless, cause to be concerned about a theory which seeks to define the moral in terms of what is "natural" for human beings. All too often what is thought to be "natural" is really only the conventional. And as feminists and other social critics point out, the conventional is often the result of bias, misunderstanding, and oppression.

If the ultimate end of our choosing is fixed by human nature, and the alternatives open to us when we seek to be virtuous are alternative ways of promoting this end, i.e., alternative ways of promoting *eudaemonia,* then the following question arises. Is Aristotle in fact advocating what we might call the *principle of eudaemonia,* as opposed to the principle of utility? And is this not a principle which can be applied, either directly or indirectly, to our actions in such a way that we have a means of determining morally right actions? For example, particular virtues like truth-telling, promise-keeping, and their ilk could be viewed as means toward achieving the ultimate end of *eudaemonia* or happiness. If this is so, then in actual fact there may be little to distinguish Aristotle's so-called "virtue ethics" from the action-centred "duty ethics" of Kant, Mill, and Ross.

Although there is some truth in this assessment of Aristotle's ethics, it would be a mistake to exaggerate it. And this is because, for Aristotle, virtuous action is not action which accords with a principle, but rather action which springs from a disposition to choose a way which lies between two extremes, the one an excess and the other a deficiency. Virtuous action lies in choosing *the mean* between extremes of behaviour one of which is a vice through excess, the other of which is a vice through deficiency. And Aristotle is clear that there is no arithmetical formula which allows us to determine with precision what lies at the mean in a particular set of circumstances. This is one reason why he says that the mean must be determined "relatively to us," and as determined not by a rule universally applicable and established in advance, but by a rule "by which a practically wise man would determine it." On Aristotle's account, there is a kind of indeterminacy in moral judgments when it comes to deciding on particular courses of action. The variable contexts of moral life prevent us from fashioning hard-and-fast rules or procedures for settling what we ought to do. The best we can do is rely on *phronesis*, our virtuous dispositions, and the examples set by paragons of virtue. We must, in other words, try under the circumstances to act as "the man of practical reason would act." This is the best that we can do. Whether this is a weakness in Aristotle's account of moral life is a good question. Perhaps the best answer is to point out that this inherent indeterminacy better reflects moral reality and the perplexing dilemmas with which we are often faced, than theories which purport to provide ready-made answers which fail to emerge when we seek to apply the theories to concrete circumstances. Is it any more helpful to be told that one must maximize utility, or seek to treat humanity as an end in itself, than it is to be told that one must seek a mean between deficiency and excess? In explicitly acknowledging that moral theory can provide only a limited amount of help, Aristotle's theory may in fact be the more honest one.

Virtue lies at the mean between the vices of excess and deficiency. Two virtues, courage and moderation (or temperance), are chosen by Aristotle to elucidate his doctrine of the mean. The accounts are perhaps dated, but they nevertheless serve to illustrate the main lines of Aristotle's thought. For Aristotle, courage is primarily a virtue of soldiers and his examples are culled entirely from the battlefield. Courage is located between the defect of fear and the excess of over-spiritedness or brashness. When the occasion arises, a courageous soldier can be counted on to subdue fear and enter bravely into the fray even in the face of death. Cowardice is the vice (defect) associated with fear. In more modern parlance, we may link it with the instinct of "flight" in the face of danger. But rashness is also a vice, in this case an excess associated with spiritedness. This vice we may link with the instinct of "fight" in the face of danger. But one can be too spirited. Soldiers emboldened by anger may rush impulsively into the fray, "blind to the dangers that await them."[26] "Right reason" moderates fear, and courage emerges as fear tempered by spirit.

Aristotle's assignation of courage to the battlefield is far too restrictive for our purposes in this book. We shall be looking for displays of courage in the more familiar domains of sickness and death. These domains are also "battlefields" of sorts in which individuals face handicap, major surgery, debilitating illness, and prolonged and painful dying. They are also domains in which health-care professionals face difficult decisions profoundly impacting upon the well-being of others, as when a physician must decide whether to recommend the termination of life-support, or whether to ask a grieving husband to allow his wife's organs to be used for implantation in others. Aristotle's ethics-of-virtue may prove helpful in such circumstances. While it may prove impossible to determine a hard-and-fast rule to answer our moral questions in such instances, it may be possible to answer the question: "What kind of people do we wish to *be* when we are faced with such circumstances?" Do we wish, for example, to be cowardly, cringing in fear in the face of death, demanding that everything conceivable be done to prolong our lives regardless of quality? Or is this an option which would not be pursued by the person of courage? Is this how "the man of practical wisdom would act," lacking in regard for others, insensitive to the fact that the resources used to prop up his life might be of more benefit to others with a more favourable prognosis? Or do we want to be courageous, moderating our fear of death and insensitivity to the needs of others as much as it lies within us to do so? In another context the relevant question might be: What kind of people do we want to be in the face of severe handicap or disability? Cowardly, living each moment in fear; or brash – at the opposite extreme from fear – living in denial, masking our true feelings from others and conducting ourselves in an unwarranted display of over-confidence or *bravado* rather than bravery? Or will we try to avoid both extremes and be courageous, striving to temper fear of death or handicap with a more reasonably nuanced and spirited response, trying to live life to the full within our disability, even though such daring involves risk? To these questions we may find reasonable answers, even if there are no rules by which they can be determined, and even if we must in the end still choose for ourselves that course of action which best exemplifies the virtuous mean.

The second virtue upon which Aristotle focuses is temperance which moderates our appetites for food, drink, and sex. One can eat too little or too much food. Aristotle designates health as the goal of eating. Gluttons are guilty of excess. They live to eat rather than eat to live. They dig their graves with their teeth. They imperil rather than preserve their health by over-eating. This is a vice of excess. The vice of defect or deficiency involves eating insufficient food in circumstances where there is enough to go around. In time of scarcity and famine, failure to eat sufficient food is not morally blameworthy. Strictly speaking, in such circumstances eating insufficient food does not qualify as a voluntary activity. Although Aristotle does not mention it, malnutrition can be caused by eating the wrong foods, not just by failing to eat enough food. One can be malnourished on a diet of soda pop and chips, or with fad diets motivated by an inordinate preoccupation with slimness. In such cases, Aristotle would attribute malnutrition to vice rather than misfortune or famine.

To be clear on Aristotle's ordering of values in this context, it must be borne in mind that while health is an immediate end of eating, it is not good in itself. Rather it is a means to happiness or well-being, i.e. *eudaemonic*, and is properly conceived only in this way. Relative to moderation in partaking of food and drink, health is a proximate end, but relative to the final end, happiness, it is *usually* a necessary means. This last point must be kept clearly in mind in medical contexts where there is sometimes a tendency to confuse means with ends. Life and "health" are important ends of human action, including medical action, but only if and to the extent that they contribute to what really counts: *eudaemonia*. When they do not, the person of practical reason and virtue will no longer see them as worthy of pursuit. The implications of this point for decisions concerning the "saving" of people who judge their lives no longer worth living are apparent and profound. Life and "health" are goods which confer rightness on the means for their achievement, but only when these contribute to *eudae-monia*.

(e) Feminist Biomedical Ethics

Many contemporary women find all the approaches to ethics outlined above to be in many respects unsatisfactory and alienating. These theories were all developed by men who, the feminists claim, inadvertently brought to bear upon their theoretical positions a number of biases and ways of viewing the world which skew the results of their analyses. The resultant theories do little justice to the moral concerns and experiences of women. Indeed, in the view of most feminist ethicists, the traditional theories "do not constitute the objective, impartial theories that they are claimed to be; rather, most theories reflect and support explicitly gender-biased and often blatantly misogynist values."[27] It would be impossible to provide a complete and fully accurate account of the important, multi-faceted themes pursued by feminist bioethicists. Instead, we will attempt, in what follows, to sketch two of the most common concerns of feminists regarding traditional ethical theories. These concerns extend to the application of the traditional theories, by ethical theorists as well as medical practitioners, to the biomedical context.

Let us begin with some important respects in which there is a natural affinity between modern feminist and biomedical ethics. First, there is the issue of power relationships. Built right into the typical biomedical context is a power imbalance between, on the one hand, vulnerable patients in need of assistance, and on the other hand, health-care workers whose knowledge, skill, and special privileges often place them in a superior position. As a consequence of this inherent power imbalance, biomedical ethicists often follow Kant's lead in stressing the crucial role of patient autonomy and control in respecting the inherent dignity of persons. Modern biomedical ethics is marked by a turning away from the paternalistic model of medicine, where doctor knows best and should be left to decide himself what is best for the patient, to models of the doctor-patient relationship which conceive of the participants as equal partners in the pursuit of the patient's wellness. The enormous weight usually placed on the necessity for fully informed, valid consent to medical procedures is an obvious fall-out of this enhanced concern for patient autonomy in the face of the typical biomedical power imbalance.

Feminists share a concern with power imbalances, principally between men and women but also between other advantaged and oppressed groups such as adults and children, the able and the disabled, and the rich and the poor. Many feminists have pointed out that both the medical profession and the field of ethical theory have historically been dominated largely by men whose perspectives may have been biased against women. Some traditional ethicists, e.g. Kant and Aristotle, thought that women have a decidedly different character from men, and are to a much greater extent than men moved by emotion as opposed to reason. In the view of these theorists, this tendency towards the emotional serves as a barrier to the level of abstract reasoning required for satisfactory moral thought. Feminist ethicists are concerned to undermine these stereotypes and to assert the equal ability of women to engage in moral thought.

Another similarity shared by feminist ethicists and biomedical ethicists is their focus on the importance of *context* in making moral decisions. Whereas traditional ethical theory tends to the abstract and general, biomedical ethical discussion tends to the concrete and the particular. It focuses on the concrete situation in which decisions affecting the health and welfare of individual patients, or groups of patients, must be made. As a result, advocates of feminist ethics quite often invoke examples and issues that arise within the biomedical context and point to the biomedical context as illustrative of the need to depart from abstract theorizing and focus on individual cases in all their particularity.

This leads to one of the most serious complaints made against traditional ethical theory by feminist ethicists. Most feminists are opposed to the search for abstract, universalizable principles and rules (or even virtues) with which to answer everyone's moral questions. The theories of Kant and Mill are often cited as illustrative of the vacuousness, indeed the perniciousness, of traditional ethical theory. In the view of many feminist critics, Kant's theory rejects the emotional, personal component of moral life in favour of the rational universalizability of individual maxims. In seeking rationally to universalize our maxims, we are inescapably led to ignore or submerge our concern for all those complex factors which *individuate* our situations and the relationships in which we find ourselves. Most importantly perhaps, in seeking such abstractions, we are led to ignore or abstract away all that makes us individual persons enmeshed in inter-personal relationships involving caring and trust. Among the factors so eliminated are the emotional bonds between people and the special concerns they have for one another, as parents, friends, siblings, and colleagues. In seeking to universalize we are, it is claimed, led to forget that most of the time we approach one another – and believe ourselves right in doing so – not as strangers subject to the same set of universalized maxims or rights, but as unique individuals in highly personal, context-specific relationships in which we have much invested emotionally. These are relationships which, by their very nature, cannot be reduced to universalized rules and principles. According to one leading feminist bioethicist,

> Because women are usually charged with the responsibility of caring for children, the elderly, and the ill as well as the responsibility of physically and emotionally nurturing men, both at work and at home, most women experience the world as a complex web of interdependent relationships, where responsible caring for others is implicit in their moral lives. The abstract reasoning of morality that centres on the rights [and duties] of independent agents is inadequate for the moral reality in which they live. Most women find that a different model for ethics is necessary; the traditional ones are not persuasive.[28]

The feminist concern for the importance of context leads in another direction as well. Feminist bioethicists argue not only for the importance of appreciating the factors which individuate one case from the other, and tie us to one another in a variety of personal ways, they also stress the importance of appreciating the wider context of decision-making. This is a context which, more often than not, profoundly influences the options available, or the options thought available, to us. Feminists look beyond the individual medical situations in which decisions are made and question the social and political institutions, practices, and beliefs that create those situations and define the available options. Consider, for example, the case of reproductive technology. Here a plethora of ethical questions arises whenever a woman requests reproductive assistance in the face of infertility. Should any woman who asks for such aid be accommodated? What if she is unmarried, a lesbian, or already has children of her own? Is it permissible to create multiple fertilized eggs when only a few will actually be implanted at any one time? If so, may some of the extra eggs be used for purposes of medical research? These questions, and many others like them, are ones which everyone in biomedical ethics will wish to address.

But feminist ethicists want to dig much deeper. They want to uncover for discussion the variety of social, political, and environmental factors which give rise to such questions and possibly frame the available answers. They wish to expose certain social factors which arguably lead many women to request treatment despite the negligible chance of success and the profound disappointment which often accompanies failure. Many argue that our conventionally accepted view of women's social role, as fundamentally involving the production and rearing of offspring, encourages infertile women to see themselves as defective and lacking in value. As a consequence, they are in effect "coerced" into seeking biomedical interventions to correct themselves. And they suffer great feelings of inadequacy and worthlessness if, as is all too common, such interventions fail to bring about the desired result. Similar points are made in relation to cosmetic surgery which, it is argued, is often pursued by women only because of the force of socially generated stereotypes of femininity which ground a woman's value in her good looks.

To sum up, feminist biomedical ethics is marked by its rejection of traditional ethical theory as far too abstract and concerned with universalized rules and principles. As such, traditional ethical theory misses out on two fronts. First, it renders irrelevant a host of individuating factors which inform our moral lives and which most of us, women in particular, consider integral to moral assessment. These include the importance of personal relationships and the emotional bonds which exist between individuals who care for one another. Second, traditional ethical theory often ignores the wider social, political, and environmental contexts in which moral questions are shaped and the available options are defined.

(7) The Language of Rights

An introduction to the basic theories and concepts of ethics would be radically incomplete without some mention of "rights." At one time it was quite natural to express moral requirements using concepts such as *ought, duty,* and *obligation.* It was in terms of the latter three concepts that the ethical theories just discussed were presented by their authors. Today, however, our moral vocabulary is dominated by the notion of rights. Instead of saying "You ought not to have done that," or "Your responsibility was to have done this rather than that," a modern person is more apt to remark "You had no *right* to do that." But rights come in a variety of different forms which are often confused with one another. In order to facilitate discussion of the moral issues raised in this book, a brief analysis of these differences follows. The conceptual map sketched is largely derivative from the theory proposed early in this century by the American legal scholar, Wesley Hohfeld and from the more recent account developed by the contemporary moral philosopher Joel Feinberg.[29]

(a) Claim-rights

Strictly speaking, Hohfeld thought, a right is an enforceable claim to someone else's action or non-action. If one has a right to X, then one can demand X as one's due. It is not merely good, desirable, or preferable that one should have X: one is entitled to it and another person, or group of persons, has a correlative duty or obligation to respect your entitlement to X. For instance, I have a right not to be assaulted by you. This entails that you are under an obligation of non-action, that is, a duty *not* to assault me. This kind of right, a claim against other people, is what Hohfeld called a *claim-right*. A claim-right is always paired with a corresponding duty or obligation which applies to at least one other person. Violation of my claim-right is always the violation by someone else of his or her duty towards me.

Claim-rights come in a variety of different forms. In sorting these out, Joel Feinberg develops three important distinctions:

(i)   in personam versus in rem rights
(ii) positive versus negative rights
(iii) passive versus active rights.

In personam rights are said to hold against one or more determinate, specifiable persons. These are determinate persons who are under corresponding or correlative obligations. For example, if Bill owes Jean a weekend at Camp David, then there is a specific person, Bill, against whom Jean enjoys his claim-right. Other examples are rights under contract, rights of landlords to payment of rent from their tenants, the right against one's employer to a safe and healthy working environment, the right against one's doctor to her best professional judgment about one's medical care, and so on. Many of the duties on Ross's list of prima facie duties could easily be expressed in terms of the correlative claim-rights. Paired with a Rossian duty of fidelity, for example, will be a claim-right against a person with whom one has made an agreement to the honouring of that agreement. That person has a duty to perform his end of the deal; you have a correlative claim-right to his performance.

Not all claim-rights, however, are held against specifiable persons. Some hold against people generally. These kinds of rights, called *in rem rights*, are said to hold against "the world at large." For instance, my right not to be assaulted holds not against any particular person or group of persons, but against anyone and everyone who might be in a position to commit such an offence against me. This includes my neighbours, people at bus stops, and surgeons who might be tempted to operate on me in a non-emergency situation without first obtaining my consent. All such persons have a correlative duty not to assault me. This latter, correlative duty, would no doubt fall under Ross's duties of non-maleficence.

Positive and negative rights form another sub-class of claim-rights. A positive right is a right to someone else's positive action. A negative right, on the other hand, is a right to another person's non-action or forbearance. If I have a positive right to something, this means that there is at least one other person who has an obligation actually to do something, usually something for my benefit. By contrast, I have a negative right when there is at least one other person who has a duty to refrain from doing something, usually something which would harm me. Depending on what it is that the other person(s) must refrain from doing, my negative right can be either passive or active.

Active rights are negative rights to go about one's own business free from the interference of others. Paired with active claim rights are duties of non-interference. Health-care professionals who complain that governments should allow them to practice medicine free from bureaucratic interference are usually asserting active claim-rights not to be interfered with or hindered in their medical pursuits. Corresponding to such rights would be a duty on the part of a government to allow health-care professionals a measure of freedom and autonomy – even when this involves such things as "extra-billing" patients over and above what is provided by a government-sponsored Medicare programme.

Passive negative rights are rights not to have certain things done to us. We might, for convenience, call them "security rights." Obvious examples are the right not to be killed or assaulted, and the right not to be inflicted with disease and injury by negligent or reckless medical staff. Health-care workers who assert a right not to be exposed to the AIDS virus also have in mind a negative, passive right. In this case it is the right not to be infected by AIDS victims. Passive rights are not rights against interference with one's own activities. Rather they are rights not to have certain unwanted or harmful things done to us.

It is worth noting that typically active rights of non-interference can be protected only at the expense of other people's passive security rights. The active right of a manufacturer to pursue a livelihood within the capitalist system often competes with the passive, in personam, security rights of workers. It also competes with the passive, in rem rights of the community or world at large not to have its environment fouled by industrial activities. In general, a key problem of moral, legal and political philosophy is how to balance active freedom rights against passive security rights. Different theories will place differing emphases on the competing rights. The resolution of such conflicts is as difficult as the resolution of conflicts among Ross's prima facie duties.

To sum up, claim rights can be either in personam or in rem, positive or negative, and if they are negative, they can be either passive or active. Correlated with any one of these rights is always a duty or obligation on the part of at least one other individual. Such rights are claims against others who are under duty to respect them.

(b) Liberties or Privileges

Sometimes the situations in which people assert rights do not involve claims against others who are under correlative obligations. Rather they involve what Hohfeld called "privileges" or "liberties." My having a privilege does not entail that others are under obligation towards me. Rather it entails only the *absence* of an obligation on *my* part. If I enjoy the privilege of doing something, then I am free or at liberty to do it (or not do it) and I do no wrong should I exercise my privilege. In short, a privilege is "freedom from duty." An example from law may help to clarify the nature of privileges.

In most legal systems there is a standing duty to provide the court with whatever information it requests. One must provide that information even if one would prefer not to. However, many jurisdictions also recognize a special area in which this standing duty does not apply. They recognize a right – a privilege – against self-incrimination. What this means is that in this special area – i.e., evidence which may implicate them in a crime – citizens are at liberty to decline the court's request. Here they enjoy an absence of duty. If the testimony in question may incriminate them, they don't have to testify if they don't want to. But notice, if I have no *claim-right* against self-incrimination, but only a privilege, then if a sharp lawyer somehow gets me to incriminate myself, he has in no way violated my rights. This would be true only if my right were a claim-right against him. Were it a claim-right, then the lawyer would be under a corresponding duty or obligation to respect a claim I would then have against him. But with privileges there are no such corresponding duties – only the absence of duty on my part. I have a freedom to act (or not to act) but it is not a freedom which enjoys the protection afforded by corresponding duties on the part of other people to respect my freedom. There is no requirement on their part that they refrain from interfering with my action or non-action.

Situations in medicine where the notion of a privilege or liberty arises are not entirely obvious at first glance. Examples can be found, however, in any situation in which some people are exempt from duties to which they would otherwise be held. Certain health-care professionals, for example, are privileged with respect to confidential information about your medical history. Access to such private, confidential information is something from which the general public is barred. The general public is under a duty to respect the confidentiality of your medical records. They have no right to these privileged items. Those who are privileged, however, enjoy a freedom from this duty. They are exempt from the general duty to keep away or to mind their own business which applies to the public at large.

Privileges also figure prominently in the doctor-patient relationship. By providing consent to surgery, for example, a patient waives his claim-right not to be "touched" by the surgeon, thereby relieving or freeing the latter from his standing duty not to touch the patient. In short, he grants the surgeon a privilege without which any act of touching would amount to assault or battery.

It is perhaps worth stressing once again that privileges are *unprotected* freedoms. Contrast a situation in which a patient grants me the privilege of examining his confidential medical records with a situation involving the Medical Officer of Health. If the Medical Officer has a claim-right to examine the files, say for purposes of tracking an infectious disease, then the Hospital (and the patient) must respect that right. They have a duty to turn the files over and do wrong if they should fail to do so. If, on the other hand, the patient simply forgets to arrange for his records to reach my hands, he has in no way violated my rights. This is because I have been granted a mere privilege, not a claim-right with its corresponding duty.

(c) Powers

Sometimes the terminology of rights is used to describe neither a claim-right nor a privilege. In some situations we have the capacity to alter existing legal or moral relationships involving rights and duties. In such cases we enjoy what Hohfeld called a normative *power*. In law, for example, we find powers of attorney which enable an agent to bring about changes in the legal relationships of his client. An agent may, for instance, be empowered to sign a contract on behalf of his client. In exercising this power, the agent imposes on his client a duty to honour his part of the agreement with the third party. He also, of course, invests in his client a right that the third party do the same. In these ways, then, the agent alters the existing normative relationships between his client and the third party.

Powers also enter into the practice of medicine. A surrogate is one empowered to act on behalf of a patient. He is able, for example, to alter the legal/moral relationship between patient and physician by consenting to surgery. In so doing the surrogate grants the surgeon the privilege of operating, relieving him of his otherwise standing duty not to invade the patient's body. Put another way, the surrogate *waives* the patient's claim-right not to be "touched." Without the exercise of this power by the surrogate on the patient's behalf, the surgeon's actions would, strictly speaking, amount to assault or battery. Of course in most cases patients themselves exercise the power of consent. But when for some reason a patient is unable to do so, the power and its exercise may fall to the surrogate, who must act on the patient's behalf. The surrogate is empowered to alter certain of the patient's normative relationships, but only when this is in the best interests of the patient.

The power to waive claim-rights will serve as a focus of attention in many of the cases that follow. In some instances, the question of who has the legal or moral power to waive patients' rights arises. In others, the issue will be whether such a power exists at all. Does anyone, patient included, have the power to waive someone's right to life?

(d) Further Reflections on Rights

While, nowadays, the rights approach to morality and ethics is most prominent, it offers no panacea for resolving moral conflicts. Instead of presenting the abortion dispute as a conflict of obligations, the obligation to protect human life (of the fetus) versus the obligation to respect human freedom (of the woman), now the tension is located in a conflict between the fetus's right to life and the woman's right to exercise control over her own reproductive processes. The same issues of comparative weight and balance remain, however.

One should be careful when encountering talk of "rights." It is always important to ask whether the right being asserted is a claim-right or a privilege, or possibly even a power. These are different conceptually and have very different implications. If the right is a claim-right, then one should ask whether it is in rem or in personam. In particular it may be crucial to determine whether the right is negative or positive. Does it require only that others *refrain* from doing something, or does it require positive action(s)? This is an important difference which figures prominently in many public debates. One famous case in which the difference proved crucial was the United State Supreme Court's decision in *Roe v Wade*. The Court ruled that every woman has a right to abort a fetus within specified limits. This was interpreted by some to mean that the Court had recognized a positive right to abortion which entailed aid and financial assistance from the government. A 1977 ruling, however, made it clear that while it was unconstitutional to prevent a woman from having an elective abortion, within the prescribed limits, women did not have a right to aid or financial assistance. In other words, *Roe v Wade* had granted only a *negative*, not a *positive*, right to an abortion.

(8) Concluding Thoughts

As the above discussion clearly illustrates, there are numerous moral theories and different vocabularies with which to express them. The question naturally arises: How should someone interested in applying the insights of ethical theory to actual practice respond to this somewhat perplexing situation? The strategies one could adopt in linking moral theory to practice are numerous and varied. Nevertheless, it is possible to isolate three basic patterns of response.

(a) Make decisions on an ad hoc, case-by-case, basis, ignoring ethical theories altogether.

Despite the undeniable importance of individual context, this is neither a promising nor an inviting option. Although there is some measure of truth in the adage that "no two cases are ever alike," it would be a mistake to exaggerate it. Any two cases will necessarily be unlike one another in many respects, but it fails to follow that they will be unlike one another *in the relevant respects*. No two murders are completely similar, but they are alike in what is often the only relevant respect: an innocent human being has been killed. If cases can be classified as being similar to one another in a limited number of relevant respects, and these cases are familiar and recurring ones, then the possibility arises of discovering moral rules and principles to govern them. We are able to fashion workable legal rules governing murder because there are a limited number of recurring, relevant aspects of murder cases which can be dealt with in simple, general rules. The same is often true with moral rules and principles. So while we must be sensitive to the importance of varying contexts, to what individuates us in our personal relationships with others, and to the dangers inherent in Aristotle's attempt to ground morality on a fixed human nature, we should also be sensitive to the importance of similarities. My relationship with my daughter is unique and special to me. It may also be very different from the relationship shared by fathers and daughters in other, more patriarchal cultures. But the relationship I share with my daughter may yet be in many ways relevantly similar to the unique, special relationships many fathers have with their daughters.

If the possibility of moral norms, and ethical theories to support and explain them, exists, then it would be counter-productive to ignore them entirely. We would have to "start from scratch" every time we had to make a difficult moral decision. This would be inefficient, to say the least, and would be a hindrance to moral understanding. Understanding the world involves recognizing similarities and differences among situations and people. Without moral rules, principles, values and virtues, and theories to generate them, we make it difficult, if not impossible, to gain moral understanding. So long as we do not claim too much for it, working with an admittedly limited theory is better than working with no theory at all.

(b) Make a firm and irrevocable commitment to a particular ethical theory.

While this option promotes single-mindedness, and simplifies our moral deliberations, it has the serious disadvantage of creating a blind spot to the possible insights of other ethical theories and approaches. It compels one to resolve all moral quandaries within the boundaries of the theory chosen and this smacks of artificiality and arbitrariness. This will be so unless one is convinced that one "knows the truth" with absolute certainty, an unlikely possibility for someone willing to ascend to the reflective level of moral thinking (see Section 3 above). Blindly committing oneself to an ethical theory or approach is no better than blindly committing oneself to a conventional rule. It is to descend to the pre-reflective level where blind acceptance replaces critical reflection and the possibility of moral progress.

(c) Allow for both fixity and flexibility.

This is clearly the preferred option. The fixity is provided by acknowledging that moral conflicts need not, and perhaps should not, be resolved within a moral vacuum, and that the application of an ethical theory with which one is not entirely happy can nevertheless shed light on the issues in dispute. It may at the very least bring some of the important considerations into relief where they may be more easily examined and discussed reasonably. Flexibility arises in acknowledging that competing theories and approaches may well offer insight as well and that one's own favoured theory is always open to improvement or, at some point, rejection. Reasonable flexibility may even lead us judiciously to extract rules, principles, or values from competing systems as determined by their apparent relevance to the case in question. It may be true that sometimes Mill provides a better answer than Kant – and that the tables are reversed at other times. It may also be true that sometimes the feminists are right in stressing the individuating features of a moral situation, features which might in some instance render the relevant issue incapable of resolution by way of a universalizable moral principle. This is not necessarily a cause for dismay, as Ross seemed to appreciate. Consider an analogous case in physics. Sometimes the wave theory provides a better account of the properties and behaviour of light than the particle theory does. At other times the reverse is true. A single, unified theory would no doubt be preferable. But till such time as one becomes available, it would be imprudent to ignore the existing theories altogether, or to subscribe to one and forget about the other(s). The same is true in moral philosophy. We must not let our failures to achieve completeness, or our failures to appreciate in all cases the full range of factors at play in particular contexts, blind us to the incremental gains in knowledge that have been made. Perhaps we would do well, in the end, to heed Aristotle's caution that "precision is not to be sought alike in all discussions. We must be content, in speaking of such subjects [as ethics and politics], to indicate the truth roughly and in outline."[30]

Notes

1   John Stuart Mill, *On Liberty*, Shields edn. (Indianapolis: Bobbs-Merrill, 1956), 56.
2   See G.E. Moore, *Principia Ethica* (London: Cambridge University Press, 1903).
3   John Stuart Mill, *Utilitarianism* (New York: Bobbs Merrill, 1957) 10.
4   *Utilitarianism*, 22.
5   John Rawls, "Two Concepts of Rules," in *The Philosophical Review*, January 1955.
6   See J.J.C. Smart and Bernard Williams, *Utilitarianism: For and Against* (London: Cambridge University Press, 1973), 10.
7   See David Lyons, *The Forms and Limits of Utilitarianism* (Oxford: Oxford University Press, 1965) where it is argued that any version of RU faithful to the utilitarian credo collapses logically into AU.
8   Immanuel Kant, *Groundwork of the Metaphysics of Morals*, trans. H.J. Paton (New York: Harper and Row, 1964), 67-8.
9   Kant, 70.
10   Kant, 89.
11   Kant, 89-90.
12   Kant, 90.
13   Kant, 96.
14   See Lloyd Tataryn "From Dust to Dust," in D. Poff and W. Waluchow, eds., *Business Ethics in Canada*, eds. (Scarborough: Prentice Hall Canada, 1987), 122-25.
15   W.D. Ross, *The Right and the Good* (Oxford: Clarendon Press, 1930), 21.
16   Ross, 13.
17   Immanuel Kant, "On a Supposed Right to Lie from Altruistic

Motives" in Lewis White Beck, ed. and trans., *Critique of Practical Reason and Other Writings in Moral Philosophy*, (Chicago: University of Chicago Press, 1949), 346-350.

18   Ross, 21.

19   Leslie Stephen, *The Science of Ethics* (New York: G.P. Putnam's Sons, 1882), 155, 158.

20   Aristotle, *Nicomachean Ethics*, translated by J.L. Ackrill (New York: Humanities Press, 1973), 1094a1-3.

21   Aristotle, 1095a16-20.

22   Aristotle, 1106b36 – 1107a2.

23   William Frankena, *Ethics* 2nd ed. (Englewood Cliffs: Prentice-Hall, 1973), 63.

24   Aristotle, 1112a16-17.

25   Aristotle, 1113b20.

26   Aristotle, 1116b37.

27   Susan Sherwin, "Ethics, 'Feminine Ethics,' and Feminist Ethics,' in Debra Shogan, ed., *A Reader in Feminist Ethics* (Toronto: Canadian Scholar's Press, 1993), p. 10.

28   Sherwin, p. 14.

29   See W. Hohfeld, *Fundamental Legal Conceptions* (New Haven: Yale University Press, 1919) and Joel Feinberg, "Duties Rights and Claims," in *Rights, Justice and the Bounds of Liberty* (Princeton: Princeton University Press, 1980)

30   Aristotle, 1094b12, 18.

Chapter 1: Doctor-Patient-Family Relationships

Case 1:1 When Physicians and Family Disagree

Mrs. François is a 63-year-old French Canadian, 5 feet in height and weighing 315 pounds.

Her case was presented to a gynaecologist as one of stress incontinence. An ultrasound of the pelvis was carried out, revealing an ovarian cyst. The gynaecologist elected to perform a hysterectomy and bilateral oophorectomy (removal of both ovaries). During the operation both the bladder and the sigmoid colon were injured. The sigmoid colon injury was a laceration in the bowel. This was oversewn. The patient was put on antibiotics post-operatively.

Six days later she suddenly developed severe abdominal pain and became hypotensive (blood pressure dropped dramatically). This occurred at approximately 11 a.m. She was transferred to the Intensive Care Unit where her blood pressure was raised with Dopamine and intravenous fluids. Because of her respiratory distress she was intubated.

As the day progressed her blood pressure rose to 100 systolic, her condition gradually improved, but she continued to be maintained on a respirator. Her pain continued and she had a fever of 37.8°C (100°F).

A surgical opinion was requested and the patient was examined by the surgeon at 6:30 p.m. An examination revealed Mrs. François to be suffering from generalized peritonitis. Her abdomen was distended, tender, and non-moving. There were no bowel sounds. The most probable diagnosis was dehiscence (splitting open) of the colonic suture line. This was confirmed by the results of a barium enema ordered earlier in the day, which revealed leakage from the sigmoid colon. In spite of all this, her general condition was reasonably stable.

Mrs. François appeared to be alert and aware of where she was; she communicated by means of written notes in a way that appeared both rational and sensible.

When Mrs. François learned she needed an operation, she refused to give consent. Even when it was explained straightforwardly and realistically that without another operation she would in all probability die, she still refused surgery. Indeed she threatened to have the police called if her wishes were disregarded, and demanded to be released from hospital.

Her family was greatly distressed, so the explanation for surgery was repeated in the presence of two family members. Mrs. François refused the operation even more adamantly.

By 8:30 pm. her husband and four children had gathered in the waiting area of the Intensive Care Unit in deep distress. They wished to consent to the operation on Mrs. François's behalf. It was explained that this could not be done since the patient was conscious and apparently competent. Her elder son, Jacques, arrived from a trip abroad at approximately 9:30 p.m. When he was apprised of the events that had taken place he declared that his mother was behaving abnormally, and insisted that she really did not understand the consequences of her refusal of surgery. When the surgeon showed reticence to operate against Mrs. François's wishes, Jacques issued the warning, "If you do not operate, you will be responsible for my mother's death and you will hear further from me."

What ought the surgeon to do?

Case Discussion

(1) The Problem

In this case the surgeon is confronted with the problem of whether to operate in a life-threatening situation against the patient's expressed wishes. To do so in absence of an overriding reason would constitute a violation of the patient's right to self-determination. A likely overriding reason would be the physician's obligation to provide the patient with necessary medical care. The physician's obligation is particularly pressing in this case because the proposed surgery falls into the category of life-saving treatment. Thus the surgeon is caught between two conflicting obligations. The first is to respect the patient's wishes and hence her right to self-determination, and the second to provide medically indicated treatment. Consider whether or not these obligations can be ranked in order of importance. How would Mill rank these in terms of utility? And how would Kant react to the suggestion that the (apparently) fully-informed, rational decision of a patient to refuse life-saving treatment can be overridden? Could a maxim which required this course of action be universalized?

(2) The Legal Crunch

Reflect on the surgeon's reticence to operate against the patient's expressed wishes in connection with the following observation: "an offensive touching or invasion of the body, if not consented to, is a trespass against the person, a battery, redressible in an action for damages."[1] This would be the case in all North American legal jurisdictions. Two reasons may be given for the physician's reluctance to operate: (a) respect for patient autonomy, and (b) fear of legal reprisals. There is no need here to settle the question of motivation. It is sufficient to note in passing that (b) is also relevant to the decision not to operate.

The son's threat, "If you do not operate, you will be responsible for my mother's death and you will hear further from me," introduces another legal pressure point. Now the physician is threatened by fear of legal action if he *fails* to operate. In (1) above the surgeon was confronted with a conflict of obligations. Now he is faced as well with conflicting threats of legal action. If he operates he may be charged with "trespass against the person." If he refuses to operate he possibly faces charges of criminal neglect.

Is there a way out of this legal impasse? Can the probabilities of legal action be ranked? For example, is the patient less likely to sue than the son? Suppose she is. Would that count as an adequate reason for overriding the patient's expressed wishes? While it might be *prudent* from the legal standpoint to take the line of least resistance, would it be *moral* to bypass the patient's right to self-determination simply because it is safer? Would it be fair to expect a physician to run the greater risk of serious legal sanction for doing what he believes is right?

(3) The Consent Requirement

One of the requirements of valid consent is that the patient be given sufficient and appropriate information to make an intelligent decision. All ethical theories, even AU, support the need for valid consent. Supporters of AU will point to the long-range damage to trust and the welfare of patients that would result were the requirement for valid consent ignored. Recall our earlier discussion of "desert-island promises." Valid consent involves two steps: (a) relevant and sufficient information must be presented to the patient, and (b) this information must be presented in a way that is understood by the patient. Determine whether these conditions have been met in this present case. For example, is there more that could or should have been done before the arrival of the son who insisted on surgery? In attempting to answer this question it will he helpful to determine whether direct or surrogate consent to surgery is appropriate.

(a) Direct Consent
Until the arrival of the son who demanded that the surgeon operate, it appears that this case was conducted on the assumption that valid consent was both possible and appropriate. In addition to the requirement to present the relevant information in a way that the patient understands, valid consent operates within the limits of legal and mental competence. Minors and mentally incompetent patients are precluded from valid consent. Two other values are also involved: (a) the need to honour the patient's expressed wishes, and (b) the need to promote the patient's best interests. Indeed the physician's obligation to provide medically indicated treatment derives from the good to be realized by meeting the needs expressed in (a) and (b).

Where the patient's expressed wishes and the promotion of his/her best interests coincide, the tension identified in (1) above, between the patient's right to self-determination and the physician's obligation to provide medically indicated treatment, does not arise.

Problems arise, however, when the patient's expressed wishes are at odds with the physician's judgment of what is in the patient's best interests. Physicians experience little or no difficulty with refusals of treatment for minor maladies. Refusal of medical interventions for serious illnesses or injuries, however, gives the health-care professional some bad moments because it involves being a party to withholding potentially beneficial treatment from a patient. Refusal to do what one can is likely to be perceived as a failure of moral duty. Furthermore, when life-saving treatment is refused, as in the present case, the patient may be suspected of incompetence. This suspicion may, of course, be ill-founded. While refusal of life-saving treatment may qualify as "eccentric" or "idiosyncratic," it need not be irrational. Consider the case of the Jehovah's Witness who refuses a blood transfusion. While health-care professionals may be dismayed at such a refusal and deem it to be unwise, nevertheless the adult patient's wishes are usually respected in such circumstances. Does the refusal of life-saving treatment in the case now being considered fall into the category of competent, though idiosyncratic, refusal of treatment, or into the category of incompetent refusal? On what basis could one tell? And if one cannot be confident of one's answer either way, then in which direction should one run the risk of error?

(b) Surrogate Consent

Scrutinize the case again prior to the arrival of the son who insisted on surgery. Do the patient's threat to call the police and her demand to be discharged from hospital give grounds for concern about her mental competence? Indications of possible cognitive disorientation came from her family. It is difficult to explain, however, why the family failed to tune in to the possibility of their loved one's disorientation before the arrival of her son. Jacques, by contrast, appears to have quickly sized up the situation, observing his mother's abnormal behaviour and her failure to realize the consequences of her actions. But even before the son's arrival, should someone not have noticed the discrepancy between the woman's willingness to submit to the first operation and her adamant refusal to consent to the second?

The patient's expressed wishes are now quickly short-circuited in favour of the patient's best interests, narrowly interpreted in terms of life-saving therapy. The short-circuiting appears to be justified, however, because the usual basis for classifying her behaviour as idiosyncratic and eccentric rather than abnormal is seriously in question. To revert to the Jehovah's Witness case again, while we may question the wisdom of Jehovah's Witnesses who refuse blood transfusions, we do not question their sanity. Their behaviour, while judged peculiar from a different life perspective, nevertheless coheres with the structure of beliefs adopted by, and behaviours acceptable to, adherents of their particular religious persuasion. With the arrival of Jacques this patient's behaviour was perceived to be out of character rather than a reflection of any customary eccentricity. If this line of reasoning is sound, then it warrants a challenge to an uncritical honouring of the patient's expressed wishes. Respect for the autonomy of individuals does not require respecting their expressed wishes if these can be shown to be seriously out of character and irrational.

With the "expressed wishes" criterion in limbo, the surrogate is forced to resort to promoting the patient's best interests. Unfortunately "best interests" is ambiguous, embracing both (a) preserving the patient's life, and (b) promoting the patient's values, which may or may not include preserving his/her life at all costs. This amounts to the familiar distinction between life and quality of life. The distinction compels us to consider whether the patient's quality of life is so diminished that death is preferable. If it is, then there may be grounds for refusing, on her behalf, a second round of surgery. If not, then ranking her best interests above her expressed wishes may be justified.

(4) Patients' Rights

Reflect next on the implications of the claim that patients have a right to refuse (even life-saving) treatment. If the patient has a right to refuse treatment, then someone (presumably, in this case, the physician or health-care giver) has an obligation to honour that right. Sometimes, however, the obligation to honour a patient's right conflicts with another obligation, namely, the physician's obligation to provide medically indicated treatment.

In an attempt to mediate between these conflicting obligations, it has been observed that the patient's right to refuse treatment is a relative right. If it were an absolute right it would "reduce medical ethics to patient autonomy."[2] May we propose a companion truth? If the physician's obligation to provide medically indicated treatment were absolute, medical ethics would be reduced to physician paternalism. Some kind of balance needs to be struck between the values in competition in these two positions. This might be the point at which one considers whether patient refusal of treatment "is the bottom line in a relationship in which the patient is entitled to exercise power," or the beginning of a dialogue in which the outcome is negotiated. Dialogue of course presupposes patient competence to give or withhold consent. In cases where competence is in doubt the dialogue then takes place between the physician and appropriate members of the patient's family.

Initially, in the present case, the physician tended to take the patient's refusal as "the bottom line" rather than as a point of departure for negotiation. Should he have explored more vigorously the reasons for her refusal of treatment rather than accept it at its face value?

Notes

1   Richard T. Hull, "Patients Rights and Responsibilities: Questions of Consent," in John Thomas, ed., *Matters of Life and Death*, (Toronto: Samuel Stevens, 1978), 279.

2   Paul Ramsey, *Ethics at the Edges of Life* (New Haven: Yale University Press, 1978), 156.

Case 1:2 Prescribing Birth Control to Minors

Brigitte Roberts is a 15-year-old who lives at home with her parents. She attends a nearby school and has become sexually active. This, and concern over a late period and a vaginal discharge, lead her to visit a drop-in clinic at the Planned Parenthood Office.

Brigitte expresses concern over her late period and a vaginal discharge, and indicates she would like to "go on the pill." She has no money to pay for oral contraceptives and does not know her parents' medical insurance number. When the question of consulting her parents is raised by the physician, Brigitte insists that her visits to the clinic be kept completely confidential.

Brigitte then confides that she has been going with her present boyfriend for six months, that he is older (19) and works at a downtown plant. They have been sexually active for four months. She has learned about birth control at school and is sure she cannot be pregnant because her boyfriend always uses a condom. Her parents think Brigitte is too young to have a steady boyfriend, but she likes him and enjoys the physical part of the relationship.

Brigitte started her periods when she was 12. They occur every 20-25 days and last 5-7 days. Her last period started about six weeks ago. There is no breast tenderness, nausea or vomiting. About a week ago, a few days after having intercourse, she noticed a vaginal discharge. It was yellow coloured, with no odour, and was not accompanied by any itchiness or soreness. She has had no abdominal pain or fever.

An examination reveals a temperature of 36.9°C (98.5°F). Brigitte's abdomen is flat, soft, and not tender to palpation (examination by touch). The liver and spleen cannot be felt, and there are no masses. The pelvic examination reveals the cervix to be pink coloured with a yellowish discharge from the os (opening). The vaginal mucosa (mucous membrane) is not inflamed. Further examination reveals the cervix to be non-tender, the uterus mobile and slightly retroflexed (tilted backwards). The uterus cannot be felt by the abdominal hand. No tenderness or masses are detectable in either adnexa (i.e. uterine appendages like the uterine tubes). A smear and culture are then taken from the endocervix, and a pregnancy test ordered.

The next day Brigitte telephones with the news that her period has started. By this time the laboratory results are back, revealing the pregnancy test to be negative. The smear, however, has shown gram negative rods in pairs and occasional gram negative diplococci, intracellular, in pairs. The culture report is not back yet.

Brigitte then reports that her boyfriend has left town after being laid off and she doesn't know where to reach him. Nevertheless, she still wishes to go on the pill.

The physician then invites Brigitte in for a follow up. Later, the results of the culture reveal she has gonorrhoea.

What should the physician do?

Case Discussion

Problems Arising from the First Visit

(1) Should physicians prescribe contraceptives to minors?

Fundamentally this is a question about the morality of prescribing oral contraceptive pills for minors. The legality of doing so is still at issue in some North American jurisdictions, but not in Ontario where Brigitte resides. There, a physician may prescribe contraceptives for minors without parental consent *if* the minor is, or is about to become, sexually active. But what is legal is not necessarily moral. While in recent years North American society has become more receptive to the idea of sexual activity among minors, there are individuals and groups who view sex outside of marriage as immoral. There are also those who believe that most minors lack the emotional maturity required for responsible sexual activity. This latter point is particularly crucial to some in light of the dangers of sexually transmitted diseases, principally but not exclusively, HIV.

In a pluralistic society one might reasonably expect to find a "live and let live" attitude. But it is seldom that easy or tidy. It is tempting to adopt the attitude that our views concerning morality and prudence are correct and quite natural to wish that they will be shared by others. It should not come as a surprise, therefore, if tensions should arise between the players in the drama presently under consideration.

(a) Brigitte and the physician at the clinic
It is possible that Brigitte's views on sex and those of the physician at the clinic might be fully compatible. But suppose they are not, or that Brigitte had gone to her family physician whose views on sexual activity among minors were in agreement with those of Brigitte's parents who were strongly opposed to such activity on moral and prudential

grounds. If they had been, then a crucial question would arise: Should Brigitte be refused her request for contraceptive pills because to prescribe them violates the physician's own conscience, or his sense of loyalty to Brigitte's parents? Would it be morally permissible, perhaps even obligatory, for the family physician to refer Brigitte to another doctor whose moral sentiments are more in accord with her own? This raises a more general question: Do physicians who have moral scruples about matters like prescribing contraceptives to minors, or about a procedure like abortion, have a moral obligation to refer them to another physician? If so, does this not impose an obligation on them to facilitate a course of action which they believe to be wrong? Assuming that they do have such an obligation, would it be a violation of their moral and professional responsibility to attempt first to persuade their patients that their proposed course of conduct is morally wrong? Or is the power imbalance between physician and patient, to which feminists have so forcefully drawn our attention, such that it would in fact be morally wrong for a person occupying such a position of power to attempt to influence the moral judgment of a patient? Especially if, as in this instance, the patient is a female minor and the physician is a male adult.

(b) Brigitte and her parents

The fact that Brigitte wishes to keep the information about her sexual activity from her parents points to fundamental differences in outlook on the morality and/or prudence of sexual behaviour among minors. Some parents are morally opposed to sex among minors, or to sex outside of marriage. Brigitte's parents may fall into one of these categories. It is arguable that prudence favours contraception for a sexually active minor in order to minimize the risk of unwanted pregnancy. But some people disagree, believing that the risks of sexually transmitted diseases are so great that it would be wrong to facilitate in any way sexual activity among minors. Providing them with contraceptive pills virtually erases the fear of pregnancy which might otherwise serve as a deterrent to sexual activity. It may encourage minors to underestimate the serious health risks involved in promiscuous sexual activity. Studies have shown that some individuals actually believe that contraceptives serve as an adequate defence against sexually transmitted diseases as well as against pregnancy.

Suppose there was reason to believe that Brigitte's parents reject both the morality and the prudence of prescribing contraceptives to minors? What weight, if any, should those views be given in this case. More precisely: (i) Whose views should take precedence? and (ii) How could we justify the preference?

(i) Whose views take precedence?
This is a difficult question to answer, not simply because of the probable conflict between Brigitte and her parents, but because the conflict occurs between adults and a minor within the context of a family relationship. Parents are not only obliged to provide for their children's necessities, they are also entrusted with the lion's share of responsibility for their children's moral education. Were this a value conflict between adults, the daughter's right to self-determination would, of course, clearly override paternalism. This is because parental status, in itself, is neither a necessary nor a sufficient condition for parents to pull moral rank on their adult children. But the situation is not so clear when there is a minor involved.

Though Brigitte is a minor, it could be argued that she is sufficiently close to legal age to warrant discretionary action on the part of the physician at the clinic. Close proximity to, or the attainment of, chronological age is, however, no infallible indicator of maturity in the sense that counts. Indeed, chronological age is not even a reliable guide to physiological maturity.

(ii) On what grounds do we justify giving precedence?
While it has been acknowledged that parental status is neither a necessary nor a sufficient condition for parents to pull moral rank on their adult children, we have seen that this is not obviously true when the children are minors. The view that parents may override their children's wishes when they judge it to be in their children's best interests to do so has at least *prima facie* plausibility.

We have supposed that the physician has good reason to believe that Brigitte's parents have views about the morality and/or danger of sexual activity among minors which are strongly opposed to their daughter's views. Should the physician (a) simply write the prescription with no questions asked? Or should he (b) insist that Brigitte talk things over with her parents before prescribing the contraceptives? If she refuses, then what should the physician do? Should he (c) undertake to act *in loco parentis* by seeking assurances of cognitive and emotional maturity before acquiescing in this particular minor's wishes? Or (d) should the physician report Brigitte's request, together with the activities which prompted it, to Brigitte's parents?

In light of such considerations, the physician who shares Brigitte's moral viewpoint might think himself justified in withholding information from the parents. He might believe that this course of action, though morally problematic, is still preferable. Would it be right for the physician to take matters into his own hands in this way? Is this one of those circumstances where it would be wrong to exploit the power imbalance inherent in the doctor-patient relationship?

(c) May the physician breach confidentiality in this case?

The confidences exchanged between patient and physician belong to the category of "privileged information." All other things being equal, the physician may not breach confidentiality. Are all things equal in the case of minors? Ideally a rational decision reached by all affected parties – patient, parents and physician – is highly desirable. But we may have to settle for less than the ideal. As a minimum requirement should Brigitte be encouraged to discuss the matter with her parents? The operative word is "encouraged" since she cannot be required to do so. Suppose she refuses to do so. Would it be morally wrong to violate Brigitte's right to confidentiality, or is this right over-ridable in such a context? Suppose it is reasonable to think that Brigitte's parents could, with a bit of coaxing, be brought to acknowledge that they are setting an unrealistic standard, and that their daughter, like many other people's daughters, may fail to achieve the ideal? They might, then, be persuaded that the use of contraceptives is morally preferable, as the lesser of two evils. Would it be right, under the circumstances, for the physician to go ahead and attempt to persuade the parents of the wisdom of prescribing oral contraceptives? Suppose on the other hand, that it is reasonable to think that Brigitte's parents could not be persuaded to adopt a more lenient stand and would in fact become alienated from their daughter if they knew of her activities. Would it be right for the physician in this instance to threaten the integrity of the family relationship by informing the parents?

Bearing the above discussion in mind, consider the following maxim: "In cases of conflict between 'mature minors' and their parents, where agreement is impossible, give precedence to the adolescent patient's informed decision, made in concert with a qualified physician, over the parents' wishes." Could this be adopted as a guiding principle in Brigitte's case? Would adoption of this maxim maximize overall utility? Would it represent a universalizable maxim? Is this the only way in which we can protect mature minors from the unwarranted paternalistic intrusions of physicians and parents?

(2) May the physician use the parents' medical insurance number without their consent?

It is one thing to withhold information from parents in order to respect the autonomy of mature minors. It may be quite another to use the parents' medical insurance number to pay for their daughter's treatment without their knowledge. The term "knowledge" is used advisedly. In Ontario, which has a government-funded, compulsory health insurance plan, physicians and medical centres bill the government directly. Consequently, Brigitte's parents would be unaware that their daughter's treatment had been billed to their number. This system facilitates prescribing the pill and treating Brigitte's venereal disease without fear of discovery. But even though it is legal to treat Brigitte without parental consent, is it moral to do so without their knowledge? Would doing so violate Kant's Categorical Imperative? Recall Kant's second formulation of the Categorical Imperative: I must always "Act in such a way that [I] always treat humanity, whether in [my] own person or in the person of any other, never simply as a means, but always at the same time as an end."[1]

A Problem Arising from Subsequent Visits

The main problem arising out of Brigitte's subsequent visits to the physician is confirmation that her vaginal discharge is a symptom of venereal disease. With the contraction of a communicable, infectious disease, the legal net tightens. While the physician may be permitted the use of discretionary powers in prescribing the pill for a minor without the knowledge or consent of parents, failure to report a case of venereal disease to the Office of the Medical Officer of Health is a punishable offence in law.

Since all persons sexually active with venereal disease remain, until cured, a reservoir of infection and a constant threat to others, treating both partners is a bona fide expression of preventive medicine. Even though it may not be possible to trace her partner, the physician has a legal and moral obligation to treat Brigitte and report this case of gonorrhoea. We have now reached the legal limits of privacy which permit us to pursue our interests and desires providing that we do no harm to others. Brigitte is now a potential source of harm to others and the physician's obligation to report incidences of venereal disease derives from the social spin-off of the doctor-patient relationship. Confidentiality now yields to public good.

How would you respond to the suggestion that since gonorrhoea is a milder form of venereal disease, curable by the administration of antibiotics, the physician should be allowed the use of discretionary powers in reporting such cases? Should we become crusaders for law reform on this issue?

One final worry deserves mention. In Brigitte's legal jurisdiction she is a minor under the age of consent. The older sexual partner could, as a result, be charged with statutory rape. Does the physician have a professional obligation to treat this information as confidential? Suppose Brigitte did not have gonorrhoea but had just come for oral contraceptives. Should the physician just turn a blind eye?

Notes

1   Immanuel Kant, *Groundwork of the Metaphysics of Morals*, trans. H.J. Paton (New York: Harper & Row, 1964), 96.

Chapter 2: Fetal Rights?

Case 2:1 When a Couple Disagree Over Abortion

Bob and Linda Thompson are a happily married, middle-class couple. Bob is a 35-year-old Associate Professor of History at the University of Central Ontario. The 32-year-old Linda has spent the past seven years at home caring for their two children, Shannon who is 7 and Shawn who is 5. Linda resigned her position as a hospital nutritionist when Shannon was born in order to provide their children with a loving home environment. Over the years Bob has also been intimately involved in raising Shannon and Shawn. The Thompsons present a paradigm of shared parenthood.

Following Shawn's birth, Bob and Linda decided not to have any more children. Now that their younger child was enroled full-time in primary school, Linda wished to resume her career as a nutritionist. Sterilization was considered, but ultimately rejected; the couple wished to leave their options open just in case they later changed their minds. Instead, Linda was fitted with an IUD.

Despite their efforts to avoid conception, Linda became pregnant. Owing to the irregularity of her menstrual cycle, and to her misidentification of morning sickness with a nasty virus, the pregnancy was not confirmed until well into the fourth month. When informed of the news, Bob was overjoyed. He really had wanted another child for the past two years, but hesitated to mention it to his wife for fear she might feel pressured to postpone her return to the workforce. But now that she was pregnant, he believed the decision was effectively "out of their hands."

Linda, on the other hand, was anything but happy and insisted on an immediate abortion. She, like her husband, had once thought abortion to be morally wrong. But the prospect of an unwanted pregnancy had caused her to have second thoughts on the matter. Putting her career plans on hold for another five years was more than she could bear.

Bob was both perplexed and angered by his wife's position, insisting that an abortion was totally out of the question. In his view, such an act would violate their unborn child's right to life. It would be an unjust killing of an innocent and defenceless human being, and would also deprive both him and the rest of their family of a welcome addition. He noted that both Shawn and Shannon had been overjoyed when he told them of their mother's pregnancy.

Linda was outraged. She was incensed that the children had been informed and strongly opposed the suggestion that the decision was anything but hers to make. Bob countered this with the claim that the decision was a family matter. Linda disagreed, arguing that abortion is a matter of personal conscience for the woman involved. No one has the right to tell a woman what is to be done with her own body, to impose his or her own moral views. She is not prepared to succumb to attempts by our male-dominated, patriarchal society to relieve women of their freedom to decide what will be done with their own bodies. Furthermore, it is not true that abortion in the fourth month amounts to killing an innocent human life. It involves at best eliminating the potential for human life – something the two of them had been doing for years by practising contraception. A four-month-old fetus is anything but a human person invested with rights which compete against those of the woman who bears it. It is, to be sure, a potential bearer of rights; but it no more has rights than an acorn has branches.

Upon hearing his wife's newly expressed views, Bob once again insisted that an abortion would violate the right to life enjoyed by their child from the moment of its conception. He suggested further that the issue could not simply be left to Linda's discretion. It is one thing to respect individual autonomy when no one but the agent herself is seriously affected by her decision. It is quite another to do so when the interests of others are at stake – including one whose very life lay in the balance. Abortion is not a "victimless crime" which can be properly left to individual decision.

The next week, Linda checked into a local clinic, and over the objections of her family, had an abortion. Was Bob or Linda right in this case?

Case Discussion

(1) Two Different Bases

Contemporary disputes about abortion tend to revolve around a conflict between two competing rights: the right to life and the right to personal and bodily integrity. Almost always, this conflict of rights is based upon competing conceptions of the fetus. There are those who view the fetus as a full-fledged bearer of rights with a moral claim to our care and respect. In their view, the life of an innocent, defenceless human being far outweighs in importance the right of a woman to control her bodily processes. Abortion, on this view, is a monstrous violation of an innocent being's right to life – it amounts to murder.

At the other extreme are those who see the fetus as nothing more than a biological organism which has yet to achieve moral standing. On this view, the woman's right to personal and bodily integrity is of paramount importance, since there is no competing moral right to outweigh it. Attempts to prohibit women from seeking abortions are viewed as unwarranted violations of personal autonomy, as impositions of other people's moral values. Feminists are particularly worried about such denials, arguing that they are the product of attempts by a society dominated by males to control the reproductive capacities of women. Keeping women "barefoot, pregnant, and in the kitchen" are the traditional means by which men have attempted to dominate women over the centuries. Seizing control from men requires, among other things, reproductive freedom, which in turn requires unlimited access to abortion on demand.

(2) Bob's Stand

Bob clearly sides with the first of the two views presented above. His position is based largely on the premise that an abortion would violate the unborn child's right to life. On the view he defends, this right exists from the moment of conception, when a unique, human life, worthy of our utmost respect and protection, comes into being. To him the right to life outweighs all other competing considerations, including his wife's "right" to decide what shall be done with her body. It is for this reason that he insists that Linda should not have an abortion. He views his intervention not as an unjustifiable infringement upon Linda's personal autonomy, but as a fully warranted defence of his defenceless child. The limits of freedom and autonomy of moral agents are reached when their exercise can harm other people. And what greater harm can there be than to have one's life snuffed out before one has a chance to begin living it?

(3) Linda's Position

Linda, unlike her husband, denies the moral standing of the fetus she carries within her womb. She is therefore led to radically different conclusions. In her view, the fetus is a *potential* bearer of rights with no claims that compete with her right to personal and bodily integrity, and with her right, as a woman, to be free of the pernicious control of patriarchal society. The only possible constraint, then, lies in the interests of Bob and their children. But according to Linda, those interests are effectively "trumped" by her right to control her own body. Since it is her body, she *alone* is entitled to decide whether or not it may be used to nurture a potential life into existence. This is why, of course, Linda resented Bob's insistence that he and the children were entitled to participate in the decision-making.

(4) Four Questions

(a) Fetus or unborn child?
As we have seen, the positions of Bob and Linda rely heavily on their competing conceptions of the fetus/unborn child. Which, if either, of these conceptions is correct? Is a four-month-old fetus a "person" in possession of moral rights which can compete with the rights of others? Or is it an unconscious being, lacking a concept of self and incapable of reason, communication, or self-motivated activity – in reality not a person at all?[1] Is it enough that such a being has the *potential* for all these properties? Or is their *actual* possession necessary? If actual possession is required, must a fetus enjoy them all if it is to have full moral standing? If not, then which ones will suffice? Another question arises: Are we confident that a four-month-old fetus is neither conscious nor self-aware? How can we tell? If unsure, must we give the fetus the benefit of the doubt? If not, why should we give the benefit of the doubt to newborn infants lacking these same properties?

(b) Who decides who counts?

According to Linda, she alone is entitled to decide on an abortion. Is this correct? Does she have an unqualified discretionary power in the matter? Or does Bob, and perhaps to a lesser extent Shawn and Shannon, have a right to participate in the decision-making process? Do they at least have a right to have their views seriously considered? Perhaps the decision should be a joint one made only after all the affected parties (except the fetus/unborn child) have been consulted. Or is Linda's stake in the decision so much higher than all the rest that the decision should be her's exclusively? Recall the feminists' contention that the cards are stacked against women's autonomy and freedom in these contexts. Does this fact provide overwhelming weight to the thesis that we must insist on a woman's complete freedom to decide in such cases?

Consider, now, how one might respond were the roles reversed. Suppose Bob wanted an abortion to permit Linda to return to the workforce but Linda wished to go ahead with the pregnancy? Would it then be fair for Linda to decide the matter herself? In our modern western societies, we expect fathers to share in the rearing of their children, a responsibility Bob had discharged faithfully, and could be expected to continue to do in the future. If we expect fathers to assume the burden of these responsibilities, is it fair to deny them a right to participate in decisions resulting in the birth of their children? Would this not be an unfair imposition? If it would, does the unfairness extend to decisions resulting in the termination of pregnancies? In such cases there would be no imposition of an unwanted responsibility. But the father may nonetheless feel that he has a serious stake in the decision. Is it fair that a pregnancy should be terminated in the face of a father's morally-based concern for the welfare of his "unborn child?" Or is the mother's right to decide of such serious social and moral importance that it must outweigh these concerns?

(c) Mother versus unborn child

So far the discussion has assumed that if the fetus is a "person" its right to life outweighs Linda's right to personal and bodily integrity. Is this assumption unassailable? Judith Jarvis Thomson thinks not. She invites you to imagine waking up one morning connected to a famous, unconscious violinist who for nine months needs the use of your kidneys to survive. The hospital's director expresses regret that a Society of Music Lovers co-opted your body for this purpose, and assures you that neither the hospital nor the violinist would have permitted it had they known. But now that the deed has been done, to unplug you would kill the innocent violinist. (Recall Bob's claim that the decision was now out of their hands.) In response to your vigorous protest, the director offers this defence of his position, "All persons have a right to life, and violinists are persons. Granted you have a right to decide what happens in and to your body, but a person's right to life outweighs your right to decide what happens in and to your body. So you cannot . . . be unplugged from him."[2] Thomson supposes that we would regard this as outrageous. But if so, then arguing by analogy, perhaps we must challenge the view that a fetus's "right" to life automatically outweighs a woman's right to control her body. Or are there relevant differences between Linda's case and the one Thomson presents? If so, are these differences sufficient to warrant different conclusions?

(d) Is there an acceptable middle way?

Linda and Bob represent two widely divergent, and extreme, views concerning the status of abortion. In the one view, the right to life trumps all other considerations. In the other, the right to personal and bodily integrity has the same effect, particularly in the oppressive social context in which many women continue to find themselves in late twentieth-century western culture. Are these really our only two choices? Or should we be prepared to *weigh* these two rights, with the understanding that each might have to give way to the other under certain conditions? In one case, perhaps, the imposition upon a woman whose life is at risk, or who has been victimized by rape or incest, would be far too great. In another, the fetus might have reached a stage in its development where its right to life overrides all other factors. Several developments have taken place which provide support for the latter possibility. Lowering the age of viability has enabled us to save fetuses at an earlier stage of development than was hitherto possible. Neonatal care transforms the fetus from "an 'abortable' product of conception" to a "cherished baby" or "patient."[3] The introduction of ultrasound facilitates the visualizing of the fetus in its individuality and reality. Ultrasound pictures amplify "the role once assigned to quickening, that moment at which a woman becomes physically aware of the growing fetus within."[4] Knowledge of fetal development renders untenable the "tissue theory" that equates the status of the fetus with that of a wart or polyp.

If we go this route of balancing the rights of the woman against those of the fetus, then we seem to lack clearly definable lines. As a result, our decisions become much harder to make in a principled manner. Is this a reason to prefer one of the more extreme views defended by Bob and Linda?

Notes

1   See Mary Anne Warren, "The Moral and Legal Status of Abortion" in J.E. Thomas (ed.), *Medical Ethics and Human Life* (Toronto: Samuel Stevens & Co., 1983), 99-106.

2   Judith Jarvis Thomson, "A Defence of Abortion," *Philosophy and Public Affairs*, 1, no. 1 (Fall, 1971).

3   Daniel Callahan, "How Technology is Reframing the Abortion Debate," *Hastings Center Report*, 16, no.1 (Feb. 1986).

4   Callahan.

Case 2:2 The Role of Chantal Daigle's Boyfriend in Her Abortion Decision

On July 26, 1989, a panel of the Quebec Court of Appeal ruled that a fetus was a "distinct human entity" with a constitutional right to life and protection under both the Quebec Charter of Human Rights and Freedoms and the Canadian Charter of Rights and Freedoms. This ruling stunned and angered members of the "pro-choice" movement and delighted those within the "pro-life" group. It represented the first case in which a Canadian court had expressly ruled that a fetus has constitutional rights.

Chantal Daigle was a pregnant, 21-year-old secretary. Jean Guy Tremblay, her former boyfriend, had asked the Quebec Superior Court for an injunction to prevent Daigle from having an abortion. Interestingly, Tremblay's Superior Court petition was filed on July 7, three days after the Ontario Supreme Court had granted an injunction in a similar case, involving Barbara Ann Dodd.[1] Quebec Superior Court Judge Jacques Viens granted Tremblay's request on July 17, placing Daigle's fetus, then about 20 weeks of age, under the court's temporary protection. Ms. Daigle filed an appeal with the Quebec Court of Appeal.

The Court of Appeal divided, 3-2, on the question whether the injunction should be lifted. Justices Bernier, Lebel, and Nichols ruled that a fetus does have constitutional rights that are not superseded by a woman's right to an abortion. Unlike his two colleagues, Nichols declined to take the step of declaring the fetus a "person," but he was happy to rule that the fetus does have rights apart from those of its mother. Justices Tourigny and Chouinard dissented, arguing that a fetus has no rights separate from its mother and that denying a woman an abortion violated the Canadian Charter of Rights and Freedoms, section 7 of which establishes the right to "life, liberty and security of the person."

On July 27, Daigle filed a second appeal with the Supreme Court of Canada asking for an expeditious decision, as the time beyond which an abortion would be dangerous was fast approaching. On August 8, the Canadian Supreme Court, on the basis of a unanimous decision, lifted the injunction. Shortly before the ruling was handed down, Daigle's lawyer, Daniel Bédard, informed the justices that his client had already ended her pregnancy. What follows are excerpts from the judgment later announced by the Court.

(1) The Judgment of the Supreme Court of Canada

The respondent [Tremblay] argues that a fetus is a "person" who has a "right to life" under the Quebec Charter [of Human Rights and Freedoms] and Civil Code ...

Insofar as Mr. Tremblay argues for the injunction on the basis of the alleged right of the fetus, it is clear that he must be acting as a representative of the fetus.

Some arguments were made concerning whether Mr. Tremblay should have standing in this respect; that is, whether he should be able to argue that the rights of another person are in danger of being infringed. In view of how this appeal will be decided this is not a crucial issue, but we note that, if the respondent's allegations of fetal rights were accepted, it would seem that he would be an appropriate person to assert such rights. As the potential father of the fetus in question, Mr. Tremblay would appear to have as much interest in the fetus and as much right to speak on its behalf as anyone, save the appellant [Daigle] ...

The respondent's argument is that a fetus is an "être humain," in English "human being," and therefore has a right to life. [This] argument must be viewed in the context of the legislation in question.

The court is not required to enter the philosophical and theological debates about whether a fetus is a person, but, rather, to answer the legal question of whether the Quebec legislature has accorded the fetus personhood. Metaphysical arguments may be relevant but they are not the primary focus of inquiry. Nor are scientific arguments about the biological status of a fetus determinative in our inquiry.

The tasks of properly classifying a fetus in law and in science are different pursuits. Ascribing personhood to a fetus in law is a fundamentally normative task. It results in the recognition of rights and duties – a matter which falls outside the concerns of scientific classification.

In short, the court's task is a legal one. Decisions based upon broad social, political, moral, and economic choices are more appropriately left to the legislature....

No cases dealing with the issue of fetal rights under the Quebec charter have been brought to our attention. The charter is framed in very general terms. It makes no reference to the fetus or fetal rights, nor does it include any definition of the term "human being."

The respondent, however, makes two arguments which are based on the text of the charter. The first argument is that a fetus simply is a human being in the plain meaning of the term…. His contention is that the word "human" is in reference to the "human race," of which the fetus is a part, and that the word "being" signifies "existing," which a fetus certainly does. Thus the respondent concludes, a fetus is a human being.

The argument is not persuasive. A linguistic analysis cannot settle the difficult and controversial question of whether a fetus was intended by the National Assembly of Quebec to be a person. The meaning of the term "human being" is a highly controversial issue, to say the least, and it cannot be settled by linguistic fiat …

In our view the Quebec Charter, considered as a whole, does not display any clear intention on the part of its framers to consider the status of the fetus. This is most evident in the fact that the charter lacks any definition of "human being" or "person."

For her part, the appellant argues that this lack of an intention to deal with a fetus' status is, in itself, strong reason for not finding fetal rights under the charter.

There is force in this argument. One can ask why the Quebec legislature, if it had intended to accord a fetus the right to life, would have left the protection of this right in such an uncertain state. As the case demonstrates, even if the respondent's arguments are accepted, it will only be at the discretionary request of third parties, such as Mr. Tremblay, that a fetus's alleged right to life will be protected under the Quebec charter. If the legislature had wished to grant fetuses the right to life, then it seems unlikely that it would have left the protection of this right to such happenstance …

The respondent argues that a fetus is recognized as a human being under the Civil Code [of Quebec]. His argument rests on two propositions: (1) that Article 18 directly recognizes that a fetus is a human being; and (2) that a variety of other articles in the code indirectly recognize that a fetus is a "juridical person," and, since juridical persons are natural persons … a fetus is a human being …

In our view, the respondent's argument ignores the words of the articles and the way in which the courts have interpreted them. The recognition of the fetus's juridical personality has always been as this court stated in *Montreal Tramways Co. v. Leveille* (1933), a "fiction of the civil law," which is utilized in order to protect the future interests of the fetus.

This is equally true in Quebec civil law. Articles 608, 771, 838, and

2543 explicitly state that, unless the fetus is born alive and viable, it will not be granted the rights recognized therein. If the fetus is not born alive and viable, the interest referred to in the articles disappears, as if the fetus did not exist ...

For all of the foregoing reasons, we conclude that the articles of the Civil Code referred to by the respondent do not generally recognize that a fetus is a juridical person. A fetus is treated as a person only where it is necessary to do so in order to protect its interests after it is born ...

While Anglo-Canadian law is not determinative in establishing the meaning to be given to general terms in the Quebec charter, it is instructive to consider the legal status of a fetus in that body of jurisprudence. It is useful to do so as well to avoid the repetition of the appellant's experience in provinces with the common law [i.e. all provinces other than Quebec].

A number of Anglo-Canadian courts have considered the status of a fetus in cases which are similar to the present appeal. These courts have consistently reached the conclusion that, to enjoy rights, a fetus must be born alive.

The argument based upon "father's rights" (more accurately referred to as potential father's rights) is the third and final basis on which the substantive rights necessary to support the impugned injunction might be founded. This argument would appear to be based on the proposition that the potential father's contribution to the act of conception gives him an equal say in what happens to the fetus ...

There does not appear to be any jurisprudential basis for this argument. No court in Quebec or elsewhere has ever accepted the argument that a father's interest in a fetus he helped create could support a right to veto a woman's decision in respect of the fetus she is carrying.

A number of cases in various jurisdictions outside Quebec have considered this argument and explicitly rejected it...We have been unable to find a single decision in Quebec or elsewhere which would support the allegation of "father's rights" necessary to support this injunction. There is nothing in the Civil Code or any legislation in Quebec which could be used to support the argument. This lack of a legal basis is fatal to the argument.

The conclusion to the foregoing discussion is that the foundation of substantive rights on which the injunction could possibly be founded is lacking. It is unnecessary to go any further in order to decide that this appeal should succeed. We therefore conclude that the appeal should be allowed.

Five Questions

Keeping in mind the preceding case of Bob and Linda, consider the following questions:

1. Should the law recognize fetuses as "persons" worthy of the law's protection?

2. Even if the law should not accord "personhood" to fetuses, should the law nevertheless take a direct interest in protecting fetal life?

3. If so, can you imagine cases where the rights of the prospective mother to determine what shall be done to her own body must give way to the interest in protecting fetal life?

4. If we suppose that no one but the pregnant woman has the right to decide whether to terminate her pregnancy, is it nevertheless true that a woman's decision to terminate a pregnancy may yet be morally wrong?

5. Assume that the previous question is answered positively. Was it morally wrong of Chantal Daigle to terminate her pregnancy in light of Mr. Tremblay's profound objections, even though she had the legal and moral right to make that decision?

Note

1   For a report of this case see *Maclean's Magazine*, July 31, 1989. The Ontario injunction was later overturned and Dodd had her abortion. A few days following her abortion, Dodd publicly declared her regret at having gone through the abortion, both puzzling and angering those within the pro-choice movement who had publicly supported her cause. Dodd claimed to have been overly influenced by this group.

Case 2.3 Protecting an "Unborn Child": The Case of Ms. G.

Ms. G. was a pregnant 22-year-old addicted to glue-sniffing and use of other solvents. She had already surrendered three children to the Winnipeg Child and Family Service and two of these children were both physically and mentally damaged from birth as a result of their mother's solvent addictions. The Child and Family Services Agency successfully sought an injunction to force Ms. G. into a treatment facility against her will in an effort to protect her unborn child. A lower court upheld the injunction, which raised the ire of many individuals, including many feminists, who argued that the woman's right to control her own body, whether pregnant or not, must be provided the strongest possible protection. It was further argued that this protection is provided by the Canadian Charter of Rights and Freedoms which guarantees every individual a right to security of the person. The Manitoba Court of Appeal agreed, and overruled the lower court's decision, ordering that Ms. G. be released from the treatment facility. The Winnipeg Child and Family Service agency pursued the case to the Canadian Supreme Court arguing that society has a duty to protect the rights and welfare of the unborn fetus. In the meantime, Ms. G. gave birth to a baby who was, by all accounts, unaffected by the mother's addiction. Ms. G. has reportedly stopped sniffing glue, is free of drugs, and is pregnant again. The Supreme Court of Canada refused to overrule the Manitoba appeal court.

Case Discussion

(1) Harming non-existent persons

As we have seen, modern controversies over abortion revolve around two conflicting rights: the right to self-determination on the part of the pregnant woman, and the right to life on the part of the fetus. As we have also seen, many deny that the latter right exists at all since they deny that the fetus is a person with moral or legal rights, including a supposed right to life. So we are left with the right to self-determination which is usually thought to trump any other considerations there might be in favour of preventing abortions. It is a crucial feature of abortion that it pre-empts the birth of a person. There is (or will be) no person who can later complain that his or her rights have been violated. This includes, paradoxically, the right to life, or perhaps more accurately, the right to be born. If there were such a thing as a right to be born, it would not be the sort of thing which a person can be denied and later complain about.

But this is not true of what we might call a "right not to be intentionally, recklessly, or negligently harmed in utero." Ms. G. gave birth to a child who does exist and who is now, arguably, in a position to complain about her glue-sniffing. This has the air of paradox. Had Ms. G. decided to terminate her pregnancy, thereby "depriving" her unborn child of life – i.e., killing her fetus – there would have been no basis for complaint. No rights would have been violated because no person would exist whose rights and interests had been thwarted. But now we do have a person. Given her decision to bring her pregnancy to term, Ms. G. seems to have placed herself in a position where she can (justly?) be criticized for harming a child to whom she could rightly have denied life. But perhaps this is not the proper way to describe the situation. It is not that she could have denied life to a child; rather it is that she could have denied *herself* the opportunity to bring a child into existence. Before the child's birth there was no child to be denied anything, including life. But given the decision to go on with the pregnancy, there will be a child, whose future rights and interests can be affected by behaviour which preceded his or her existence. Hence, the possibility of harming a non-existent child.

(2) A Further Paradox

Suppose that it is true that a yet-to-be-born child has a basis for later complaining of harm caused by his mother's actions while in utero. Suppose, further, (a) that if X has a basis for complaining about harm caused by Y; and (b) X is unable to act on his own behalf; then (c), all else being equal, it is permissible (perhaps mandatory) for a third party, Z, to act so as to protect X from Y's harm. We are now faced with further questions and further paradoxes. Is it morally permissible for Z to act on X's behalf *before X comes into existence*? Or must Z await X's birth before actions can be taken? In Ms. G.'s case the ruling of the higher courts was that birth must first take place. We saw the same position articulated in the Chantal Daigle case, where the Supreme Court of Canada noted that recognition of the "fetus' juridical personality has always been ... a fiction of ... law ... which is utilized in order to protect the future interests of the fetus." As the court further noted, this is certainly true under the Civil Code of Quebec which explicitly states that "unless the fetus is born alive and viable, it will not be granted the rights [it] recognize[s] ... If the fetus is not born alive and viable, the interest referred to ... disappears, as if the fetus did not exist...." Again we have the air of paradox. We can act to protect the interests of an as-yet-to-born child only after it has been born. The harm we seek to prevent is caused by actions which precede her existence, and can be prevented only at that time. We cannot do so then, but must wait till it is too late, at which point the best we can do is attempt to ameliorate the harm and seek compensation. Whether this is a rationally and morally acceptable stance for the law to take is open to question. Once the decision has been made to carry a fetus to term, then it is arguable that society has a right to protect its interests before its birth. That the fetus has yet to be born, or may yet be aborted, it still seems reasonable to insist on some measure of protection.

(3) A Slippery Slope?

In its attempt to come to grips with Ms. G.'s case, the Supreme Court of Canada placed a great deal of emphasis on the perils of the slippery slope whose logic is as follows.

Assume we are now in state A. Should we take a certain step and alter our attitudes, practices or principles, we will land in State B. State B is desirable – or at the very least not undesirable. And so were we confident that we could remain in State B we would have no objection to taking the proposed step. But the slope is slippery, and so we are not confident that we could remain in State B. Any step towards B will inevitably or probably cause us to land in State C, which unlike State B, is clearly undesirable. We have reason, then, not to take the step towards B. The slippery slope argument has, then, two pivotal claims:

i.   Movement to State B will inevitably or probably cause movement to State C; and

ii. State C is for some reason undesirable.

In response to the request that the Court intervene to prevent Ms. G from carrying on with her glue-sniffing, Chief Justice Antonio Lamer reportedly said, "If limits on freedom can be imposed for sniffing glue, can they also be imposed for smoking or drinking? And how much would warrant intervention? Can a pregnant woman work in a place where there is a lot of smoke?"[1] Lamer is clearly expressing concerns about sliding down the slippery slope. He is concerned that if we prevent pregnant women from sniffing glue, State B, we will end up preventing women from drinking alcohol and from inhaling second-hand smoke, State C. The relevant questions now are: Is there a principled way to stop the slide down the slope? Is there no way in which the Courts could distinguish glue-sniffing from smoking cigarettes or from imbibing the occasional social drink? And would it really be undesirable for us to take steps to prevent such things? Perhaps it *should* be illegal to abuse alcohol or smoke tobacco while one is pregnant.

(4) Reproductive Freedoms

It is at this point that many will balk at any such suggestion on grounds of the right of a woman to determine the course of her own pregnancy. Most people would object, for example, to the suggestion that parents should be charged with unlawfully subjecting their minor children to second-hand-smoke. The same would apply if the children in question have yet to be born. But the fact that we are talking about children who have yet to be born implicates the issues discussed earlier in the previous two cases. If, as many feminists argue, the right of pregnant women to control their own bodies is one of the most fundamental rights in the fight for gender equality, then perhaps we should tread lightly on any attempt to curtail that right. Whether the potentially great harm caused to an unborn child by her glue-sniffing mother is of sufficient weight to override these concerns for reproductive freedom is a question which must be faced. According to the Canadian Royal Commission on New Reproductive Technologies, the answer to this question is No.

> Society has an interest in promoting the health and well-being of the fetus, but not at the expense of the basic components of the woman's human rights – the right to bodily integrity, and the right to equality and human dignity. To coerce and compel ... is also unlikely to be effective in protecting the fetus. The instruments available ... are blunt and unsuited to the goal of promoting anyone's well-being.[2]

Do you agree with the Commission's conclusion?

Notes

1   Janice Tibbetts, "High Court Struggles with Case of Glue Sniffing Mom," The Canadian Press, June 19, 1997, as printed in *The Niagara Falls Review* of that date.
2   *Report of the Royal Commission on New Reproductive Technologies: Summary and Highlights* (Ottawa: Canada Communication Group Publishing, 1993).

Chapter 3: Pre-Natal Screening and Non-Treatment of "Mentally Disabled" Newborn Infants

Case 3:1 Should Fetuses With "Milder Defects" be Aborted?

Mrs. Brown, aged 42, presented herself for amniocentesis in the second trimester of her pregnancy, to determine whether she was carrying a child afflicted with Down's Syndrome. The test was negative on Down's Syndrome but chromosomal analysis revealed an abnormality. Her child-to-be had 47 instead of 46 chromosomes, confirming the presence of Klinefelter's Syndrome.

Normal human beings have 46 chromosomes in each body cell. Eggs and sperms have half that number. Gender is determined by the sex chromosomes (X and Y). Females have two X chromosomes and males an X and a Y. Errors in division can result in an extra chromosome in each cell. This is what happened in the present case. Instead of the pattern XY, Mrs. Brown's future child exhibited the pattern XXY.

This chromosomal aberration can express itself in the following ways:

(1) Physical symptoms
   (i) tallness
   (ii) low fertility (oligospermia)
   (iii) infertility (azoospermia)
   (iv) breast enlargement (correctable by surgery)

(2) Mental and behavioral symptoms
   It was once believed that there was a higher frequency of mental retardation among individuals with Klinefelter's Syndrome.

Follow-up studies have not supported this view, though a tendency to behaviour disorders has been confirmed. This takes the form of difficulty in adapting to the environment. Some sufferers from Klinefelter's Syndrome respond by being overly aggressive, others by being overly withdrawn. A careful use of testosterone has been effective in handling the behaviour problems, particularly during adolescence.

When this information was presented to Mr. and Mrs. Brown, Mr. Brown was not particularly upset. The problems likely to be encountered did not appear to him to be unmanageable. Furthermore, this was their last chance at having a child of their own. Given their ages, adoption also appeared to be out of the question. So if his wife felt the same way, he was in favour of her carrying the child to term.

Mrs. Brown did not receive the news with the same degree of equanimity as her husband. Two things rankled her. First, the presence of the extra X chromosome became indissolubly associated in her mind with "female engendering chromosome." She feared that her child would suffer sex-identity crises. Second, despite assurances that the old association of mental retardation with Klinefelter's Syndrome was unfounded, she could not convince herself that her child would not be retarded. Because of these unshakeable fears, Mrs. Brown was inclined to favour a therapeutic abortion. As she put it, "It's not as though our marriage is on the rocks. We don't need a child to save our marriage. While a child would enrich our relationship, we don't need one to cement it. I know my husband will be supportive of me whatever decision we finally make." She pleaded for more time to arrive at a decision.

It was explained that, given legal constraints on termination of pregnancy, she only had ten days at the outside in which to make up her mind.

What should Mr. and Mrs. Brown do?

Case Discussion

Women of Mrs. Brown's age are at high risk for chromosomal aberrations. While one of the main reasons for offering amniocentesis is the detection of Down's Syndrome, chromosomal testing frequently reveals other genetic anomalies, some more severe than Down's Syndrome, others less.

(1) Relevance of Severity of Defect

One fact inhibiting the decision-making process in this case is that the probable consequences of Klinefelter's Syndrome are relatively less severe than those of Down's Syndrome. Furthermore, Down's Syndrome is itself a milder species of genetic aberration. It should be made clear that these comparisons are based upon degree of impairment, and not on differences in the emotional responses of parents to the prospect of impairment to be sustained by their would-be children, however mild.

Indeed, this way of expressing the matter raises two questions: (i) is such a comparative scale possible? and (ii) even if it is, should it influence the decision whether to abort a mildly affected fetus? The first question may be answered affirmatively. We do consider anencephaly to be more serious than a cleft palate, and spina bifida with associated hydrocephaly as more serious than Down's Syndrome. Ranking in terms of departure from a norm is common to medical practice, testifying to the existence of more objective criteria than the emotional responses of prospective parents to the news that their child-to-be will not be "normal."

The answer to (ii) is much more complex because of the presence of the word "should," which carries moral overtones. Why would one appeal to the comparative scale in the first place? Is it to dissuade a woman carrying a mildly affected fetus from having an abortion? If so, how could the scale be employed to achieve this end? Acknowledging that the scale is not very precise (agreement at the extremes would be easier to achieve than in between) the mild and severe cases as just noted are easier to identify and reach agreement on than the intermediate cases. This being so, the scale could be invoked to proscribe abortions in the case of mild handicaps and permit them in the case of severe handicaps. The other cases would call for an exercise of judgment.

But perhaps the point of specifying mildness or severity of handicap is to facilitate an autonomous, informed decision. One could imagine the information that one is carrying a severely handicapped fetus being used either to seek an abortion or to prepare oneself psychologically and in other ways to accept and care for such a child.

Whether the same flexibility is warranted in the case of mild disabilities is moot. The decision to abort is likely to meet with stiff opposition. Is the abortion of mildly affected fetuses universalizable

(Kant)? Can we elevate the termination of pregnancy in such cases to the status of public policy? And even if we could, could we do it without assigning a disproportionate value to "normalcy"?

(2) To Inform or Not to Inform?

Consider next quite a different issue – the proposal that in cases of mild "defect" parents ought not to be burdened with information because, in their distraught condition, they may blow it up out of all proportion. In this case why not fall back on therapeutic privilege? Since physicians may, arguably, sometimes withhold information from patients if they deem it to be in their patients' best interests, why not withhold information about their prospective child's affliction from Mr. and Mrs. Brown? Such a course of action would, of course, have to be justified morally. And any plausible justification would have to take into account the following observations:

(i) The only known defect associated with Klinefelter's Syndrome is sterility. Statistics indicate, however, that sterility, attributable to a variety of causes, is on the increase. Consequently, Mr. and Mrs. Brown's child will not be unique in this regard.

(ii) Tallness is a greater problem for females than males.

(iii) The earlier hypothesis of a connection between Klinefelter's Syndrome and mental retardation has been successfully challenged. The I.Q. of those affected ranges from 85-140.

(iv) Not all sufferers from Klinefelter's Syndrome have enlarged breasts. Furthermore, if this condition should occur it can be remedied by corrective surgery.

(v) Behaviour problems, *if* they develop, may be helped by the judicious use of testosterone, which boon is not open to parents of "normal" children who develop behaviour problems.

(vi) A number of worries have been eliminated in the testing process. Mrs. Brown is not carrying a eunuch (missing all or part of the genitals), a hermaphrodite (half male, half female), or a child with Down's Syndrome.

Putting all this together, few other women carry children with such a catalogue of things to reassure them. So why burden Mrs. Brown with the shadows of things that only *might* be? In trying to make a decision in this case the following factors must be taken into consideration: (1) the relevance of the adage "ignorance is bliss" to the patient's perspective; (2) the limits of paternalism from the physician's or counsellor's vantage point; and (3) respect for the patient as a person and in particular, in this case, for the patient's right to know the results of the chromosomal analysis and to make fully informed decisions about her medical care. Would failure to inform Mrs. Brown fail the test provided by Kant's Categorical Imperative which requires that we treat others as *autonomous* agents, capable of self-directed, rational action? Would this be to subject Mrs. Brown to the will of another? Recall Kant's warning that there can be nothing more dreadful to a rational creature than that her actions should be subject to the will of another.

Items (iv) and (v) from the above list add yet another dimension to the decision-making process. Earlier we discussed the problems posed by acknowledging the relative severity/mildness of disability. Reflection on (iv) and (v) now compels us to think about the morality of aborting a fetus in which the most serious defects can be remedied. In this connection one also thinks of other reparable defects like cleft palate or hare lip. Ought there to be any constraints on a woman's moral freedom in such circumstances, even if, in the end, those constraints must be self-imposed and it would be wrong for the state, or her physician, to impose them upon her? Does the fact that some "defects" are reparable or remediable have any relevance for her decision? If not, why not?

(3) A Life Worth Living?

From what has been said earlier it may be inferred that Klinefelter's Syndrome is not to be ranked among the more serious of genetic defects. Dr. George Torrance has devised a series of criteria for identifying cases in which the quality of life is so poor that death is deemed preferable.[1] He covers a range of physical and role functions, and physical and psychological health states. Measured by Dr. Torrance's criteria, Mr. and Mrs. Brown's child, were it born, would enjoy a high level of quality of life. He would be mobile, with complete control over bodily functions. Furthermore, Klinefelter's Syndrome is consistent with well adjusted males and presents no serious health problems in itself.

The limitations of this assessment, however, must be acknowledged. It focuses on the distinction between mild and serious defect, and then seeks to offer criteria for determining when the quality of life correlated with the defect is so poor that one may affirm, "This person is in a state of life worse than death." Torrance's criteria were designed primarily to assist decision-making in cases involving severe defect, and are thus of limited relevance in cases such as this. Nevertheless, they compel the reader to consider the importance of severity of "defect" to the decision-making process in the Brown case, and offer more "objective" criteria for identifying severe defects.

The term "objective" is important because, if regarded as valid, Torrance's criteria offer an alternative to parents' perceptions of the mildness or severity of disabilities or other "defects." The question that now arises is whether or not *policies* governing abortion or the non-treatment of infants should be geared to the parents' threshold of tolerance or intolerance of imperfection. Is a "threshold criterion" morally defensible, or should one aspire to greater "objectivity" (along Torrance's lines) in making life-and-death decisions involving others, particularly those as vulnerable as handicapped newborns or, arguably, children who have yet to be born?

(4) Dealing with "Irrational" Fears

How do we deal with what appear to be Mrs. Brown's irrational fears? From the evidence it is reasonably clear that Klinefelter Syndrome sufferers do not undergo any sex identity crisis, nor are they at risk for mental retardation. Is counselling appropriate in such circumstances? Does its appropriateness in turn depend on the nature and objective of the counselling? If the point of counselling is to provide adequate information for the couple, particularly Mrs. Brown, to make an informed decision, then it is clearly unobjectionable. Even if they do not particularly like what patients might do with the information they provide them, health care workers are morally obliged to provide all relevant information to their patients in order that they can make an informed decision. If, on the other hand, the point of counselling is to persuade Mrs. Brown that her fears are ungrounded and do not therefore warrant her decision to have an abortion, this could be perceived by others as coercive. Would it be coercive if her fears are demonstrably irrational? If not, then are Mrs. Brown's fears "demonstrably irrational?" Or are they irrational only from the perspective of individuals who believe that the risk of mild, and largely correctable, "defects" is well worth taking? If it is irrational to want a guarantee of a "perfect child," how is this irrationality to be demonstrated?

Consider now one last complication. Maximum freedom of choice for women such as Mrs. Brown requires that her wishes, and not the claims of a fetus, even if only mildly affected, are the bottom line. Not all agree, however, that a woman's moral freedom over her own body is *absolute*.[2] The question then remains, "If Mrs. Brown's freedom is to be moderated in favour of fetal claims, on what basis are these claims to be established?" Must we accept the view of the courts that the fetus has no legal (and moral?) standing till such time as it is born?

Notes

1   George W. Torrance, *et al.* "Application of Multi-Attribute Utility Theory to Measure Social Preferences for Health States," *Operations Research*, 30:6, November-December 1982.

2   See the three preceding cases.

Case 3:2 Should Treatment be Withheld from Patients With Severe Mental Disabilities?

Baby Girl Q was born to a 22-year-old mother who normally worked as a high school teacher. She had been married for two years; two previous pregnancies had resulted in a miscarriage and in the premature delivery at 27 weeks of an infant who died in the first 24 hours of life.

At 24 weeks of pregnancy, the mother-to-be was admitted to a local hospital with ruptured membranes. Her family doctor recommended that she be referred to the tertiary-care hospital 50 miles away where, as he said, the infant would have the best possible chance. However, after having a brief conversation with the family doctor, the mother decided to stay in the community hospital where she could be close to her husband and her own parents. Twenty-four hours later she went into rapidly progressive premature labour and delivered a baby who weighed 800 grams and who received aggressive resuscitation.

The baby was transferred to the tertiary-care neonatal Intensive Care Unit. When she was collected by the transport team, she was cold, with severe respiratory distress despite attempts to keep her ventilated.

When the baby was admitted to the neonatal Intensive Care Unit, a resident rather angrily said, "This baby would have been far better off delivered in a tertiary-care centre, and I feel it's unfair that the baby has suffered as a result of her mother not taking the doctor's advice."

At 12 hours of age, the infant had a dramatic deterioration with a fall in blood pressure and a fall in haemoglobin. Ultrasound examination of the head showed that substantial bleeding had occurred in both cerebral ventricles. By this time, the mother had also been transferred to the tertiary-care hospital. The medical staff were therefore able to meet with both parents and explain to them that the baby had deteriorated seriously. When asked what her chances were, they told the parents that the baby had a poor chance of survival and that even if she lived, there was a very high risk that she would develop hydrocephalus and suffer severe mental disability. They also mentioned that if the baby survived, there was a risk of oxygen damaging the lungs and causing problems which would be present for the first years of life, although they might eventually disappear completely.

The information resulted in the following responses:

The mother said (in tears), "I so desperately want this baby, and I really have every faith in God that Susie is going to make it. You must make sure that you give her every possible chance."

The father said, "I am frightened and confused. If she survives and is handicapped, my wife will have to stop working and I don't know how we will manage without her salary. The problems likely to arise and effort that will be necessary may endanger our marriage. Anyway, is it really fair to the baby to carry on treating her?"

The resident later commented, "Her outlook is really bad and I certainly wouldn't like to grow up as a handicapped, retarded, blind child. Are we being fair to her and are we being fair to ourselves? We are always being told how expensive this unit is, and look at how much it will cost if this baby is kept alive and requires long term institutional care!"

The paediatrician replied, "We must be clear about one thing. This little girl is not brain dead and we cannot stop her treatment on those grounds. Nor is she inevitably going to die in the very near future, which would be a further reason for stopping intensive care. I estimate that she has a 50% chance of survival. If she does survive she has a 50% chance of suffering severe mental disabilities, a 25% chance of being normal, and a 25% chance of being mildly disabled. By mild disability I mean, for example, some degree of cerebral palsy that would allow her to attend a normal school and to lead a reasonably normal life. Further, if we stop the ventilator, this doesn't guarantee her death. There is a chance that she might survive and possibly in even worse condition than she would be with continued intensive care. Now, who is going to make the final decision?"

Case Discussion

(1) Mother's Desires versus Child's Best Interests

The mother expressed the wish to remain at the Community Hospital to be assured of her family's support. Does this wish conflict with the best interests of the soon-to-be born child, which might be better served at the neonatal unit fifty miles away? The term "interests" is chosen deliberately. We are dealing with a yet-to-be born child who at this stage is not a person who has *wishes* which could be respected. Recall the earlier case of Ms. G. whose decision to sniff glue during her pregnancy was considered by the courts to be immune from state intervention. Recall, also, the puzzles that arose when we considered how best to conceptualize situations where the rights of individuals are (arguably) compromised by actions which occur before they are even born. These same puzzles emerge in this case. Does this mother-to-be have a moral right to threaten the best "interests" of her yet-to-be born child by declining the doctor's advice to move to the tertiary care hospital? Does her child, now that it is born, have a ground for claiming that her rights were violated by her mother's conduct? Or is the fact that there was no child when these decisions were taken absolve the mother of all moral responsibility?

The decision to move or stay, and later to treat or not to treat, may reflect (a) the parents' wishes or (b) what is best for the infant once it is born. These, of course, do not necessarily coincide. As we saw in the preceding case, some parents have a low threshold of tolerance of disability, while others, like the father in this case, are fearful of the impact a disabled child may have on the marriage relationship or on the economics of the family. Because (a) and (b) do not always coincide, the courts intervene sometimes on behalf of the child and overrule (a) in favour of (b). At the very least, they are prepared to do so once a child has been born.

In reflecting on this case, consider the relevance of the distinction between (i) the care to which the newborn infant is entitled, and (ii) the ultimate custody of the child. This distinction allows for the provision of medically indicated treatment *now* without committing the parents to the ongoing care of the child. Health-care professionals are enabled to initiate treatment *now* and parents to explore *later* the institutional alternatives to caring for the child themselves. This route is somewhat easier to take for Canadians than for some parents in the United States, since the costs of institutionalization are covered in Canada by a mandatory, state sponsored, medical insurance scheme rather than being borne by the parents.

While court intervention to force a move to the tertiary-care hospital would not be warranted in this case, the distinction between (a) and (b) is relevant nonetheless. In electing to remain at the Community Hospital was the woman acting on the basis of selfish or irrational motives? Perhaps this judgment is too harsh, but it is prompted by two worries arising from the apparent inconsistency between the mother's decision not to move to the tertiary care hospital for the necessary care and her later directive to give her baby every possible help. Wouldn't giving her child every possible chance have required that she follow her family physician's initial directive? Can she now be morally blamed for failure to do what was best for her child?

The answer to this question hinges, in part, on whether the expectant mother had truly grasped the seriousness of the situation. We must now consider the "informed" part of valid consent. Here the situation is complicated by the fact that there are, arguably, two patients – the woman and her (yet-to-be-born) baby. In cases where surrogate consent concerns another without profoundly affecting the surrogate herself, the decision is simpler. But here, two lives are closely entwined and the surrogate's decision will have a profound effect not only on her child-to-be, but also on the woman herself.

(2) Patient and Family Physician Interactions

If the woman failed to realize the probable seriousness of the consequences of her decision to remain at the Community Hospital for her child, can the ensuing course of events be attributed to a failure of the family physician to meet a prime requirement of valid consent? Even if the family physician could not override the woman's wishes, should not the urgency of the situation have been described more forcefully? Given the gravity of the case, was not more than a "brief conversation" required? A consultation with a specialist at the tertiary-care hospital could have strengthened the family physician's hand in effecting a transfer to a tertiary-care facility. If, in response to a stronger plea, backed by relevant information, the woman had still persisted in remaining at the Community Hospital, she might then be justly accused of putting her own negotiable interests ahead of the less- or non-negotiable interests of her soon-to-be born baby. But perhaps there is a limit beyond which forceful stressing of facts merges into coercion? Is this less a worry when someone else's future interests are profoundly at stake?

At the tertiary-care hospital the tensions emerge at different levels.

(3) Interactions Between the Parents

Following the birth of her child, the mother expressed the wish that the baby be given every chance, whereas the father questioned the wisdom of treating the child. The *family's* quality of life would likely be affected by loss of income and feared strain on the couple's relationship. While important, these are really things the father wishes for his wife and for himself. His concern for the baby is expressed in the question, "... is it really fair to the baby?" This is ambiguous. Is it unfair because the baby will probably be disabled, or because it will be reared in an unstable marriage relationship, or both? Are such considerations relevant to a decision to withhold life-saving treatment? Is there any yardstick by which to measure (a) the value of the *baby's life* versus the value of the *parent's quality of life*, and (b) the value of the *baby's life* versus the value of the *baby's quality of life*?

The difficulty posed by (a) points to the need for a sounder basis for making decisions than the wishes of the parents taken in isolation, even when parents happen to agree. There is a demonstrable need for a process of consultation in which the solemnity of our commitment to human life and the exceptional nature of deviation from it are both preserved. Distraught parents may be incapable, at least temporarily, of making a fair decision unclouded by the uncontested perceptions and self interests of one party.

Comment on (b) will follow discussion of the paediatrician's remarks.

(4) Interactions Between the Parents and the Health-Care Professionals

(a) The resident's response
The resident's remark that treatment is not fair to the baby may be intended to focus on the baby's quality of life, an issue which will be considered presently. His remark, "I certainly wouldn't like to grow up as a handicapped, retarded, blind child," raises the question of the relevance or adequacy of our personal preferences in making life and death decisions affecting others. While it certainly indicates what the resident would like for himself, it could be counterbalanced, if not cancelled out, by the testimony of disabled persons who achieve a meaningful life within the limits of their disability.

The resident's remark is skewed in another direction as well. It expresses an unwarrantedly pessimistic prognosis compared with that of the paediatrician, who predicts that if the child survives, she has a 50% chance of being severely disabled, a 25% chance of being mildly disabled, and a 25% chance of being "normal." Furthermore, there is no guarantee that if she is not treated she will die. She could survive in a worse condition than she would be in if intensive care were to be continued. The resident, of course, may still regard these odds as unacceptable, but at least we now operate with a more accurate account of them. Viewing the odds as unacceptable, however, may still amount to a subjective judgment based on the resident's personal bias and not necessarily on one calculated to promote the best interests of this disabled infant.

The second worry expressed by the resident concerns the high cost of caring for severely disabled infants. Is this not, properly speaking, a macro-ethical worry that has no place in *clinical* decision-making at the bedside? Is the appropriate response to the resident, "A physician at the bedside must not think like a policy maker?" Or does this merely allow one to "pass the moral buck"?

(b) The paediatrician's response

The usual prerequisites for non-treatment, either brain-death or terminal illness, are acknowledged by the paediatrician. Susie does not meet either of these criteria. All other things being equal she should, therefore, be treated. But are all other things equal?

The major disagreement between the paediatrician and the resident arises over the prognosis. The paediatrician's estimate of Susie's prospects, while sombre, is more optimistic than the resident's. (Indeed the resident's readiness to stop intensive care borders on a medical pessimism that would let life go when it is burdensome or frustrating.) But the paediatrician is clearly no more a medical vitalist – prepared to sustain life without any regard whatsoever for its quality – than is the resident.

The difficulty with such decisions is that they have to be made in the semi-darkness of ignorance of outcome. Generally, such decision-making occurs within a spectrum of possible outcomes. At the extremes of the spectrum the decisions tend to be black or white. Physicians usually do not agonize very long over whether to treat anencephalic infants. Nor do they experience great difficulty in aggressively caring for those suffering from mild or reparable defects. But between these extremes there is a grey area in which the decision-making process is much more difficult. Susie's case falls within this area. A 50/50 chance of severe disability weighs heavily in the calculations of Susie's parents. How should they balance the 25% chance of normalcy and the 25% chance of mild mental disability against the 50% chance of severe disability? Or how should they weigh the value of a life with severe or mild disability against non-existence? Does it make any sense at all to say that one would be "better off" dead? Eliminating the person who is affected removes the person of whom one can say, "She is better off."

The question of whether Susie's life takes precedence over her quality of life is perhaps difficult to answer at this juncture in the decision-making process. Without life, quality of life cannot enter into the reckoning. Hence the "sanctity of life" sentiment asserts that life is non-negotiable. If later, however, the quality of the life saved should turn out to be abysmally poor, the earlier decision might be regretted and the question of non-treatment will have to be faced all over again. We should only have succeeded in putting off the evil day. This would be a relevant consideration if the life-and-death decision down the road were inevitable. But it is not. If Susie survives there are, it must be remembered, three possible outcomes: (1) severe mental disability, (2) mild mental disability, and (3) "normalcy." The tension between sanctity and quality of life, and the need for the life-and-death decision associated with it are likely to recur only in connection with (1). Is it morally right to withhold Susie's treatment because of the *possibility* that (1) may occur? Is it right to "play the odds" with someone else's life? If we think not, would it make a difference if we *knew* that (1) would occur? Decisions such as these are very difficult and raise a whole host of further issues. These will be explored more fully below in chapter 8.

Chapter 4: Medical Intrusion Into Human Reproduction

Case 4:1 Difficulties with Therapeutic Donor Insemination

Marie (27 years) and Jim (29 years) are an unmarried couple from Waterloo who have lived together for six years. For five of those years Marie has desperately tried to become pregnant. Both want a child very much.

After three years they were referred by their general practitioner to the fertility clinic at a nearby medical centre. Although there was a waiting list and it would take about nine months for an appointment, Marie and Jim put their names on the list.

When their turn finally came round, testing revealed Jim to be suffering from oligospermia (low sperm count). Several unsuccessful attempts at artificial insemination homologous (AIH, insemination with the partner's collected semen) prompted the physician to suggest therapeutic donor insemination (TDI).

Both Marie and Jim, who had been following media coverage on the topic, expressed several reservations about pursuing the TDI option. What would be the legal status of their child? While the Ontario Law Reform Commission had recommended that consenting partners be afforded the status of legal parents, their proposal does not have the status of law. Related to this worry was the question, "Who is the father of a child so conceived?" Can the law by legislative fiat replace the genealogical criterion of parenting with social criteria?

Furthermore, as Roman Catholics, Jim and Marie had some moral reservations about TDI. Hadn't they read somewhere that TDI is a form of adultery and an unnatural intrusion into human reproduction? And what about the possibility of innocent incest? Isn't it possible that their child might meet another TDI child with the same "biological" father? If so, wouldn't their child be at greater risk of genetic aberrations?

Finally, Jim expressed mild concern over the prospect of his partner being impregnated with another male. He said, "I hate to admit it, but, in a way, a child conceived by TDI would be a constant reminder of my "inadequacy.""

Under these conditions, should Jim and Marie be provided with TDI?

Case Discussion

While current biomedical attempts to bypass human infertility are new, the *principle* of intervention is ancient. Witness the age-old practice of concubinage, in which half of the child's genetic make-up derived from the "surrogate" wife. To be sure, the modern modes of intervention are much greater in variety and sophistication. Nevertheless, it would be a mistake to think that they represent a novel foray into wholly uncharted territory.

Jim and Marie's case involves two modes of artificial reproduction: TDI and AIH. Others are:

(i) "in vitro fertilization" or "test tube fertilization," which involves the fertilization of an ovum previously extracted from a woman (not necessarily the woman who will bear the child) and its subsequent transfer to a woman's uterus;

(ii) "in vivo fertilization," in which a woman is artificially inseminated and the embryo removed and transferred to the uterus of another woman;

(iii) surrogate motherhood, which involves the use of one of the previous interventions to produce a pregnancy in a woman expected to surrender the newborn child to another person (or persons).

Objections to these artificial procedures fall under two headings. First, there are those which apply, in principle, to any artificial intrusion into human reproduction. These apply to AIH as much as to surrogate mothering. Then there are those objections which centre on specific aspects of one or more of the available means. Take AIH versus TDI. Some are opposed only to the latter on grounds that it, unlike AIH, violates the sanctity of the family unit by introducing a donor into the relationship.

(1) Objections in Principle

(a) The Natural Law Argument

Artificial reproduction separates procreation from the act of sexual intercourse. As such, it has been condemned as a violation of the natural order. It is difficult to appreciate the force of this argument, however. Most medical interventions are interferences with "natural" processes of bodily deterioration or malfunction. If we condemn biomedical endeavours to overcome the natural impediments of infertility, must we also condemn eye glasses as "unnatural" attempts to bypass myopia? If not, what distinguishes the two cases?

(b) The Argument from Unknown Risks

Yet another source of concern is the threat of unknown physical harm to both mother and child. Risks to the woman can arise from the surgical operations involved in in vitro fertilization and from the possibility of ectopic pregnancy. In relation to the child, attention has been drawn to the death rate among early embryos and the possibility of induced congenital abnormality. However, the currently available evidence suggests that the risks are minimal. Nevertheless, the question remains as to whether we should obtrude in these ways when little is known of the long-term effects of our interventions. Consider in this regard the use of oral contraceptives. It was well after its introduction as a common form of birth control that researchers discovered their potentially lethal side effects. The same was true of thalidomide. Is the desire to have a newborn child sufficient to outweigh these concerns? To be sure, the prospective mother, if fully informed, willingly assumes the risk of unknown harm. But the same cannot be said of her prospective child. If that child should suffer the ill effects of artificial procreation, could he rightfully complain of negligence? Or would the child have no grounds for complaint whatsoever? Consider the following argument.

(c) The Gift of Life Argument

1. It is always preferable to exist rather than not to exist. (The gift of life is the greatest gift one can receive.)

2. Any child conceived by artificial means would not have existed had some such means not been pursued.
3. Therefore, artificial reproduction is morally permissible, regardless of any risks to the child.[1]

How might one respond to this argument? Are there circumstances in which it really would have been better had someone not been born or subjected to the risks involved in his conception? Do these questions even make sense? Is there something conceptually wrong in attempts to compare existent states with non-existent ones? Another question: Is it morally permissible to employ a means of artificial reproduction when the known risks are greater than those involved in some other, possibly less effective, means? If not, does this reveal a serious weakness in the Gift of Life Argument?

(2) AIH and TDI

AIH has one advantage over TDI: children born of this procedure share genetic links with both parents. In AIH the child's social parents are identical with its genetic parents. With TDI, however, this is true only of the mother. This separation of biological from social parent, which to varying degrees is also present in the other forms of artificial reproduction, brings with it a whole host of concerns. Many of these are expressed by Jim and Marie.

(a) The Legal Status of the Child
In many jurisdictions, the legal status of the social and biological fathers is unclear. For purposes of maintenance, succession, and so forth, the law has traditionally taken "father" to mean "biological father." In the American case, *C.M. v C.C.*,[2] the semen donor, in this case known to the recipient, was held liable for child support. In Ontario (the jurisdiction in which this case occurred) a gift to the "children of X," where X is the husband of a TDI recipient, would not include the TDI child. And the semen donor's bequest to his "children" would theoretically include that child.[3] The situation with Jim and Marie is even worse. Anyone born in Ontario to a married couple is *presumed*, for legal purposes, to be the child of the husband. This presumption, it should be added, is rebuttable by "any person having an interest,"[4] including a sperm donor or a husband in the event of contested paternity. With unmarried couples, however, the

situation is very different. There is no such presumption and the male partner could not be recorded as the child's father unless he falsely declared paternity. His only legal recourse, then, would be adoption, and there is some question whether his unmarried status would render him ineligible. Other jurisdictions, on the other hand, have seen the folly in this situation. In Quebec, for example, "When a child has been conceived through artificial insemination, either by husband or by a third person, with the consent of both consorts, no repudiation or contestation of paternity is admissible."[5] But Ontario has no such provisions, and so Jim's status as legal father would be very much in doubt. These legal doubts bring the possibility of serious psychological and social harm to the child, both in its family and in society. Are these risks acceptable?

(b) A Form of Adultery

Jim and Marie raise the question whether TDI is a form of adultery. Normally, of course, adultery can occur only within the context of a legal marriage. But Jim and Marie consider themselves committed "in fact" if not in law and so the possibility of adultery looms very large in their thinking. Nevertheless, their concern seems without solid foundation. Adultery is a violation of a special trust between two people, not a purely biological matter having to do with the artificial union of genetic materials.

(c) Innocent Incest

A second concern voiced by Jim and Marie is the possibility of innocent incest: children of the same donor unwittingly entering a reproductive relationship. The offspring of such an "incestuous" relationship would have a greater chance than normal of suffering genetic aberration. "There is a one in sixteen risk of the expression of any recessive gene carried by the father."[6] The possibility of genetic defect is nothing to be taken lightly. But the chances of innocent incest are extremely small and could be rendered virtually nonexistent by legal limitations on the number of times a donor can be used. Many infertility clinics already observe such limits voluntarily.

(d) Psychological Harm

Many people regard TDI as "the introduction of a third party into what ought to be an exclusive relationship."[7] This intrusion is viewed by some as morally repugnant in and of itself (c.f. the discussion of

TDI as adultery). Others see a serious threat to the stability of family relationships. For instance, some claim a greater chance than normal that a TDI child will be unloved. It is suggested that the social father will not see the child as his own and will act accordingly. The resultant impact upon the child and the family could be severe. If true, this worry provides a powerful objection to the use of TDI in the present case. Recall Jim's concern that a child conceived by TDI would be a constant reminder of his "inadequacy." Whether or not one views such concerns about infertility as the product of Jim's "macho" hangups, the fact remains that those feelings are real and could plague the familial setting. Is it right that a child should be born into such a setting?

In answering this question consider the claim by Kraus and Quinn that "the available evidence concerning the psychological and social effects of TDI is largely impressionistic and no comparative studies appear to have ever been done." "For what it is worth," they claim, "the evidence is generally favourable to TDI and studies indicate remarkably good psychological outcomes."[8] The authors go on to point out that the only documented difficulties relate to the emotional attitudes of the mother towards the unknown donor. One study of a group of such mothers indicated that all had actively to suppress fantasies about the donor, and one-third were preoccupied with his looks and personality. Another study reported a number of failures in which the wife became "infatuated with the unknown donor and changed her attitude towards the husband, even to the extent of leaving him."[9] Whether these possible effects are sufficient to warrant a ban on TDI is left to the readers' informed judgment.

(e) Donor/Recipient Linkage

A further issue surrounding TDI is the degree of "linkage" between donor and recipient. Suppose Marie conceives a child through TDI. Should that child have access to information concerning his or her birth? Should knowledge of the donor's identity ever be revealed to the recipient child even if the donor insists on anonymity? If not, should the recipient at least have access to the anonymous donor's medical history or to medical information gathered in the process of donor screening?

Most fertility clinics have attempted to implement a system which links donor and recipient without violating anonymity. At McMaster University's Infertility Centre, semen donor files are kept separately from recipient files and coded differently. Access to both sets of files is restricted to the Director of the Infertility Centre and the Chief Executive Officer of the hospital. All parties are informed of the existence and nature of the linkage system. This seems an acceptable compromise between the need for linkage and the desire of donors, for both legal and psychological reasons, to remain anonymous.

(f) Eligibility Criteria

A final source of concern is eligibility for TDI. If TDI is provided *at all*, should it be provided *to all*? If not, then what selection criteria should we adopt? Should access be restricted to legally married couples who suffer from infertility? If not, should it be open to lesbians or single women who may not wish to pursue natural means of reproduction? Should it be available to mildly retarded couples or those whose finances are unsettled?

Marie and Jim are unmarried, but their relationship seems stable and loving. Would a refusal to provide them with the desired services amount to discrimination, to denying them a generally available medical benefit on irrelevant grounds? Would it be to treat a piece of paper as if it somehow transformed two people into suitable parents? The Ontario Law Reform Commission seems to have thought so. They recommended that "stable single women and stable men and women in stable marital or non-marital unions should be eligible to participate in an artificial conception program."[10] In their view, the important considerations are the physical and mental health of the prospective parent(s) and the child. Marital status is relevant if and only if it in some way bears on these factors.

Notes

1 A similar argument might be made in relation to the earlier case of Ms. G. whose glue-sniffing put her unborn child at risk of severe disability.

2 152 N.J. Super. 160,377 A.2d 821 (New Jersey Juvenile Court, 1977).

3 Ontario Law Reform Commission, *Report on Human Artificial Reproduction and Related Matters*, 64.

4 *Children's Law Reform Act*, R.S.O. 1980, c. 68.

5 B.M Knoppers, "The Legitimization of Artificial Insemination: Some Social and Legal Issues," Family Law Review, Vol.1, no.2, 1978.

6 Michael D. Bayles, *Reproductive Ethics* (Englewood Cliffs, N.J.:Prentice-Hall, 1984), 21.

7 *Report,* 144.

8 J. Kraus and P.E. Quinn, "Human Artificial Insemination: Some Social and Legal Issues," in J.E. Thomas (ed.), *Medical Ethics and Human Life* (Toronto: Samuel Stevens & Co., 1983), 160.

9 Krauss and Quinn.

10 *Report,* 158.

Case 4:2   The Legality and Morality of Surrogate Motherhood

Jane and Tom Saunders have been happily married for seven years. Jane is a 35-year-old corporate lawyer and Tom a 33-year-old accountant with a large firm. Last year Jane became seriously ill and had to undergo a hysterectomy which left her infertile and incapable of bearing children. This was a serious blow to the Saunders, who had planned to have a child now that their careers were fully established.

Adoption was considered but rejected for three reasons. First, Jane and Tom really did wish to have a child of their own. Secondly, they were loathe to face the several years of waiting normally involved in adoption and felt that their best "child-rearing days" might then be over. Thirdly, they had become aware of another option which struck them as preferable: surrogate motherhood. This procedure would involve another woman capable of conceiving and bearing a child. She would be artificially inseminated with Tom's sperm, bear the child, and upon birth surrender custody to Tom, the biological father. Jane could then become the child's legal mother through ordinary adoption procedures. As for the surrogate, the Saunders had to look no further than Tom's secretary Alice, who said she would be willing to serve in that capacity. Alice is a divorced 27-year-old mother of two who could use the extra money. The Saunders agreed to pay all of Alice's medical costs, the salary she would lose while on maternity leave, plus an extra $10,000 for her time and effort.

Jane drew up a formal agreement which was signed by all three parties. In return for her reimbursement, Alice agreed (a) to abstain from sexual intercourse between the time of insemination and the birth of the child; (b) not to abort the child without the consent of both Jane and Tom; (c) to maintain her health; (d) to refrain from smoking, consuming alcohol, or taking illegal drugs; and (e) to surrender custody of the child to Tom.

Of course for the arrangement to work, Alice needed to be artificially impregnated with Tom's sperm. The trio therefore approached a local fertility clinic and asked the staff to perform the TDI. They refused, suggesting that the use of surrogate mothers is unethical.

Case Discussion

Surrogate motherhood has sparked enormous public concern and controversy. Governments, medical associations, philosophers, physicians, psychologists, sociologists, and law reform commissions from all over the world have condemned the practice as a threat to legal, social, and moral values. The legislative assembly of Victoria, Australia went so far as to prohibit surrogate motherhood and impose a penalty of up to two years imprisonment. In 1985 the Ontario Law Reform Commission somewhat cautiously recommended against an outright ban.[1] Instead, the Commission called for the creation of a new body of statutory law to legitimize and regulate the practice. Their recommendation was not implemented. The more recent Canadian Royal Commission on New Reproductive Technologies strongly recommended against legalization of surrogate motherhood.

> Our review of the evidence shows that the potential benefits to a few individuals are far outweighed by the harms to others and to society. Commissioners believe strongly that preconception [i.e. surrogate motherhood] arrangements are unacceptable and should not be encouraged. Preconception arrangements commodify reproduction and children, they have the potential to exploit women's vulnerability because of race, poverty, or powerlessness and leave women open to coercion...The most appropriate ways to discourage commercial preconception arrangements are by criminally prosecuting those who act as intermediaries, and by making payments for preconception arrangements illegal.[2]

At present, surrogate motherhood is in a state of legal limbo in most jurisdictions.[3] In Ontario (where Jane, Tom, and Alice live), surrogate agreements are not prohibited by statute, except to the extent that they might violate section 67 of the *Child Welfare Act*, which proscribes payments in connection with the adoption of children. Nevertheless, they would probably be judged "illegal and unenforceable at common law as being against public policy."[4] At best, they would be declared null and void and the surrogate would simply remain the legal mother. Upon proof of paternity, the donor father could be declared the legal father, but the surrogate agreement itself would in no way entitle him to the child. Like any other father, he would be required, in the event of dispute, to apply for custody under the Children's Law Reform Act. And, as with any custody determination, "the issue would be determined according to the best interests of the child."[5] That the surrogate had agreed to surrender custody rights would have no legal force whatsoever.

(1) Why Surrogate Motherhood?

Surrogate motherhood does have its attractions. Jane and Tom, like many other couples in their situation, desperately want a child of their own. With surrogate motherhood, they at least get the next best thing: a child which is genetically related to Tom and in whose gestation and birth Jane can be closely, if only vicariously, involved. The time factor is also important. Both the Saunders, in their mid-thirties, do not wish to wait several years to adopt a newborn child. It would be a cruel twist of fate were they "penalized" for taking their parental responsibilities seriously. Had they gone ahead and conceived a child before their careers were established (and as it turned out, before Jane's illness) they could have had a child of their own.

(2) The Disadvantages

(a) Buying and Selling Babies

Despite its attractions, many people are worried about surrogate motherhood. Most objections revolve around the payment which is almost always involved. The Saunders, it will be recalled, agreed not only to pay Alice's medical costs and lost salary, but to provide her with an extra $10,000 for her time and effort. Alice would in effect be renting her uterine capacity to another party. This strikes some as an affront to human dignity and integrity. In renting her body, Alice would allow herself to be used by others as a mere means to their own ends.

One might ask however, whether this really is so objectionable. Professional athletes, for example, sell their skills, and to some degree the use of their bodies, to owners. Surgeons, auto mechanics and gardeners do much the same thing. Are these people guilty of violating human dignity? If not, then what distinguishes them from Alice?

A related objection is stressed by feminists: surrogate motherhood invites the exploitation of disadvantaged women and serves to create a class of surrogate child-bearers. One might ask in this regard whether Alice had been exploited by the Saunders. Not only did she need the money badly, she was also Tom's secretary. How might this bear on the voluntariness of her offer? Suppose, on the other hand, that the fertility clinic had cited the exploitation of Alice as their reason for refusing TDI. Could Alice rightly complain that she, a disadvantaged woman, was being unjustly denied a golden opportunity to improve her lot?

It has also been objected that "surrogate motherhood degrades the child for whose conception and transfer [of custody] money is exchanged, by treating him or her like a commodity."[6] Those who offer this objection often note that selling existing children is condemned both morally and legally in all civilized jurisdictions. It amounts to slavery, they claim; the child is treated as a piece of property to be purchased in the marketplace.

It is this powerful objection which causes the most concern among those who oppose surrogate mothering for pay. According to Michael Bayles, however, their concern is misguided. "What is being bought and sold," Bayles argues, "is not the child but the surrogate's services or the rights and responsibilities which constitute the parental role.[7] Since the bundle of parental rights does not include those of property, the child is not being treated as property. The child still has any rights vis-à-vis the parents that other children have, for example, the right not to be abused. Thus, the child is no more a slave (who lacks such rights) than other children are."[8] Whether this argument succeeds in defusing worries about baby-selling is left to the reader to decide.

(b) Physical and Psychological Risks

Payment aside, surrogate motherhood may involve undue risks to the psychological and physical well-being of both mother and child. The mother of course, runs the normal physical risks of pregnancy. But these are no greater than in normal pregnancies and provide no objection to surrogate mothering. Psychological and emotional risks are another matter. Being forced to surrender one's newborn child could be traumatic to many surrogates, some of whom may have grossly underestimated the impact of "mother/child bonding." The spectre of our wrenching a newborn infant from its mother's arms in fulfilment of a contract is more than most of us could tolerate. It is for this reason that many have recommended careful screening of surrogates, and why some would deny permission to any woman who has yet to bear a child. It is vital that the surrogate enter her agreement with both eyes open.

Possible risks to the child must also be mentioned. Some have speculated that there is risk to an unborn child in being carried by a woman whose character is such as to allow her to surrender her baby upon birth. Alice agreed to a set of conditions bearing on the health of the fetus she would carry, conditions with which most natural mothers would willingly comply out of love for their child. But can such compliance be expected of surrogate mothers who may be "in it for the money?" Should we be prepared to gamble in this way with the physical and psychological welfare of children? Should we entrust their welfare to women who lack the emotional bond which ordinarily ties the expectant mother to her fetus? Recall Aristotle's point that right actions flow from the right dispositions, which he called virtues. If, we are to ensure that the surrogate does not suffer the emotional trauma of surrendering a child against her will, must we insist on surrogates with an emotional makeup which renders that unlikely? If we do, then perhaps we will end up restricting the role of surrogate to women whose dispositions might well lead them to underestimate the importance of the fetus's interests? Do we have here a catch-22? If we seek surrogates of the appropriate disposition, we threaten the interests of the fetus. If, on the other hand, we seek to safeguard the interests of the fetus by restricting surrogacy to women whose emotional bond to the fetus will lead them to serve its interests, we threaten the interests of the surrogate: such a person will likely find it traumatic to relinquish her baby.

Consider now the possible psychological damage to the child of a surrogate arrangement upon hearing of the circumstances surrounding its birth. Would the child suffer the same effects as those adopted children whose abandonment by their natural parents results in a feeling of worthlessness?

(c) The Compliance Problem
Given the present state of local law, the "contract" between Alice and the Saunders probably has no legal force. Should either party violate the agreed conditions, the courts could not, therefore, be relied upon to force compliance. The law's impotence in these matters raises several possible difficulties which cannot safely be ignored. Here is but a small sample:

(i) Alice, like Mary Beth Whitehead, could refuse to surrender custody.[9] The impact of a long, drawn-out custody battle and its eventual resolution could prove devastating to all concerned.

(ii) The child could be born disabled, prompting the Saunders to reject it.[10] Alice might be left with a child she could ill afford to raise even with Tom's financial support.

(iii) There could be disagreements about whether Alice had been careful enough with her health or that of the fetus. These too might prompt the Saunders to reject the child should it be in some way "undesirable."

(iv) Were a problem to develop during pregnancy, strong differences of opinion might arise over the advisability of an abortion. Suppose the Saunders wished the fetus aborted because of Down's Syndrome but Alice did not.

(v) Serious difficulties could emerge should either of the Saunders die before the child was born. Alice might again be left with a child she could not properly raise.

Many of these compliance problems can of course be eliminated with legislation. But such legislation does not yet exist and so they must weigh heavily in our decision-making. Whether they, in addition to the other difficulties explored above, are sufficient to justify the clinic's refusal of TDI, is a question best left to the reader's informed judgment.

Notes

1 Ontario Law Reform Commmission, *Report on Human Artificial Reproduction and Related Matters*, 1985.

2 Royal Commission on New Reproductive Technologies, *Summary and Highlights* (Ottawa: Canada Communication Group, 1993), 19.

3 For a useful overview of how Western legal systems have responded to the practice, see The Ontario Law Reform Commission's *Report*, 221-9. Legislation addressed specifically to surrogate motherhood has been enacted in the state of Victoria in Australia. The *Infertility (Medical Procedures) Act* 1984 seeks to discourage surrogate motherhood through a series of prohibitions in relation to it and by specifying that surrogate motherhood agreements are legally void. In England and the United States, attempts by parties to use existing legislation and case law to achieve the objectives of surrogate moth-

erhood agreements have largely proven unsuccessful.

4 *Report,* 220.

5 *Report,* 220.

6 *Report,* 230.

7 Bayles refers the reader here to Lawrence A. Alexander and Lyla H. O'Driscoll, "Stork Markets: An Analysis of 'Baby-Selling'," *Journal of Libertarian Studies,* 4, no.2 (1980), 174-5.

8 Michael D. Bayles, *Reproductive Ethics* (Englewood Cliffs, N.J.: Prentice-Hall, 1984), 25.

9 An important battle was fought in 1987 in a New Jersey courtroom between Mary Beth Whitehead and Elizabeth Stern over a 10-month-old baby Mrs. Whitehead bore and refused to relinquish to Mrs. Stern and her husband, who had a contract with her to produce a child. William Stern, the biological father, pressed the courts to set a precedent and to enforce a contract in which they commisioned a child from Mrs. Whitehead for a fee of $10,000 (US). The court eventually ruled in favor of Mr. Stern.

10 Such a case occurred in the United States. For a discussion of the Malahoff/Stiver case, see *Time,* September 10, 1984, 53.

Chapter 5: Research Involving Human Subjects

Case 5:1 Using Infants in Medical Research Projects

The following proposal was submitted to the Medical Research Committee at Weetabix Medical Centre:

> We [a group of researchers] wish to conduct the following study on infants in our intermediate care nursery. On six infants we wish to compare the ventilatory response to low oxygen concentration (15% inspired oxygen) for five minutes and then repeat the experiment following the injection of Naloxone. Naloxone is a safe drug used for many years in the resuscitation of newborn infants who are depressed from opiates administered to the mother. The rationale for the study is as follows:

> Newborn infants have a response to hypoxemia (deficiency of oxygen in the bloodstream) which is quite the reverse of that in an adult. When adults are low in oxygen they breathe more deeply. Infants breathe more shallowly. We hypothesize that naturally occurring opiates (endorphines) are responsible for this paradoxical response. If this is true the response will be reversed by the administration of Naloxone. If this hypothesis is confirmed, it has very important implications for the management of children with apnoea (episodic cessation of breathing) of prematurity and with apnoea of infancy. It also has implications for the causation of sudden infant death syndrome.

If you were a member of the Research Ethics Committee would you lend your vote to the approval of this proposal?

Case Discussion

(1) The Dilemma of Experimental Medicine

The medical profession has, among its principal obligations, the duty to cure as well as the duty to improve the power to cure. This dual obligation reflects the therapeutic and research thrusts of the "medical art." The dilemma of experimental medicine is that there is often a tension between the need for scientific investigation to improve the effectiveness of treatment and the patient's claim to care. Because more effective medicine is acknowledged to be a good, it confers a *prima facie* rightness on the research necessary for its achievement. Since, however, human beings must be respected as persons, they may *not* be reduced to the status of experimental materials. Thus human inviolability functions as an effective brake on our zeal for knowledge in contexts involving human subjects.

Therein lies a difficulty. If respect for persons, perhaps based on Kant's deontological ethics, is ranked above the obligation to improve the power to cure, perhaps based on a more utilitarian approach, the pace of research may be effectively slowed down. If, on the other hand, the ranking is reversed and the experiment becomes all important, human beings may be reduced to the status of experimental materials. The moral result will be violation of Kant's Categorical Imperative which prohibits using people as mere means to the ends of other people. This violation may well be inevitable, though perhaps justifiable, when no benefit to the patient, other than the satisfaction of helping others, will accrue from the experimental measures.

(2) Controlled Clinical Trials and Valid Consent

Within the tradition of Nuremberg and Helsinki, valid consent is a necessary condition for the ethical conduct of clinical research. Although the proposed trial we are considering raises the issue of valid surrogate consent for infants in an experimental context, let us explore first the broader requirements of consent to participate in clinical trials.

(a) Ethics of Experimental Design
It is generally agreed that the following requirements are essential if experimental design is to qualify as ethical. There must be:

(i)   either genuine promise of treatment where none presently exists or genuine doubt about the efficacy of present treatment where it does exist
(ii) a clearly formulated hypothesis of the form: "If we wish result x, procedure y is a means to its probable achievement"
(iii) a protocol calculated to confirm/confute the hypothesis
(iv) a favourable risk-benefit ratio
(v)   adequate monitoring of research
(vi) adequate evaluation

In addition,

(vii) the researcher should *not* be the person recruiting subjects

(b) Ethics of (Direct) Valid Consent
It is generally agreed that the following are requirements for direct valid consent:

(i)   voluntariness
(ii) responsibleness:
    (1) legal competence
    (2) mental competence
(iii) understanding: adequate information must be *presented to* the patient/subject so that it is *understood* by the patient/subject
(iv) confidentiality
(v)   a right to withdraw

(c) Surrogate Consent to Experimental Procedures
It is widely agreed that the following are the conditions for valid surrogate consent in an experimental context:

(i)   proper identification of an eligible surrogate: *either* nearest relative *or* court appointee
(ii) qualifications of surrogate:
    (1) responsibleness:
        (a) legal competence
        (b) mental competence
    (2) understanding: adequate information must be *presented to* the *surrogate* so that it is *understood* by the surrogate
    (3) role of surrogate:

(a) to implement the dependent person's previously expressed wishes
(b) to promote the dependent person's best interests
(c) to ensure that confidentiality is maintained where relevant
(d) to exercise the right to withdraw the subject from a research project if deemed appropriate

Where 3 (a) and 3 (b) are in conflict, as in the case of direct consent by a competent subject, 3 (a) may override 3 (b) on grounds of individual autonomy and the fact that mental competence is compatible with idiosyncrasy and eccentricity. Clearly 3 (a) is inoperative where the subject's previous wishes are now known and, for example, in the case of children or severely and congenitally mentally-disabled individuals. In such cases the surrogate must base consent to an experimental procedure on what is judged to be in the best interests of the subject, i.e. must operate exclusively on the basis of 3 (b). Controversies can of course arise with respect to what 3 (b) requires in such cases.

(3) Surrogate Consent For Infants in Controlled Clinical Trials

With these matters behind us we are now in a better position to consider what ought to be done in the present case. When making decisions on behalf of an infant we are clearly in a situation in which appeal to the patient/subject's previously expressed wishes are inapplicable. Hence we are committed to making a judgment about their best interests. Other factors too must be taken into account:

(a) Therapeutic Versus Non-Therapeutic Research

Instinctively, one feels more comfortable when "volunteering" infants for novel medical procedures if the research is potentially beneficial for the patient/ subject. The research proposal we are now considering, however, is potentially therapeutic for future sufferers rather than for the subjects themselves. The direct object of the study is the knowledge to be gained, and this raises the spectre of treating these infants as a mere means to gaining knowledge that will benefit others. To be sure the knowledge sought is important – a more effective means of treating premature babies suffering from apnoea, and the provision of information about the causes of sudden death. But the bottom line is whether we may "volunteer" infants for experimental procedures designed to benefit future sufferers farther down the line.

Should this concern about treating infants as means rather than as ends have the force of proscribing *all* non-therapeutic research on infants? Certainly it would be hard to get general agreement on such a proscription. Witness the following: "Although the permissible consent to treatment for minor children is limited to procedures that are not detrimental, there is no requirement that the procedures actually benefit the child. It is sufficient if it is for the benefit of a third party."[1]

But if the proviso "it is sufficient if it is for the benefit of a third party" is acceptable, even with the qualification that the procedure must not be harmful to the subject, how would we resist the conclusion that consent should be automatic? There is an ambiguity lurking behind the word "automatic" in this question. It may mean (i) that the consent requirement should be abandoned entirely, thereby relinquishing control to the physician-researcher; or (ii) that consent should be automatically given by the surrogate. Neither meaning affords much protection to the infants in question or preserves a "voice" for them, albeit the voice of a surrogate who speaks on their behalf. How would we justify such treatment of infants, when we do not consider consent to harmless research to be "automatic," in either sense of that term, in the case of adults? If we are not prepared to bypass consent to experimental procedures involving adults, why should we do so in the case of infants? Would different treatment of infants not only invalidate genuine surrogate consent but also be unjust?

(b) Basis for Surrogate Consent for Infants

Determining the grounds for surrogate consent for infants is controversial. In specifying the role of the surrogate we saw that the requirement of "honouring the patient/subject's expressed wishes" is irrelevant to the present proposal. In experimental contexts surrogates are expected to act on behalf of subjects incapable of giving consent. Inaccessibility to previous wishes and the inapplicability of the obligation to "promote the subject's best interests" leaves only the protective umbrella of the ethical requirements for experimental design. If we refuse to let those requirements carry the day, on what grounds should surrogate consent be given or withheld in the present case?

It is interesting to note that in the case of direct consent, meeting the requirements of experimental design may not substitute for seeking the subject's valid consent to an experimental procedure. This is so even if refusals to participate fall into the category of "idiosyncratic" or "eccentric." Insistence on the consent requirement for conscious, competent subjects, however, is predicated on the distinction between the subject's desires or preferences and his/her best interests. The subordination of interests to desires or preferences is allowable in certain circumstances because they are the subject's own desires or preferences. In exercising surrogate consent on behalf of infants it is tempting to base that consent on the *surrogate's* desires and preferences rather than on the infant's. To do so, however, would disqualify the surrogate's decision as a genuine substituted judgment.

(c) Benefiting Actual Patients vs. Manipulating Statistics

It may be objected that the envisaged group of beneficiaries in this proposal (future sufferers) is a statistical creation rather than a genuine class. So, submitting actual sufferers to a "risky" experimental procedure to benefit, as yet, non-existent future sufferers is unacceptable. Consider the impact of this objection on the conduct of medical research if the sentiment it embodies were to be universalized.

Note

1   Joseph E. Magnet and Elke-Henner Kluge, *Withholding Treatment From Defective Newborn Children* (Quebec: Brown Legal Publications Inc. 1985), 52.

Case 5:2 Research Involving Alzheimer Patients

Ann Wilson was the director of St. Mary's Nursing Home, a large regional centre for the care of elderly people suffering from Alzheimer's disease, a form of senile dementia. One day Ann received a telephone call from Dr. Sandra Selleck, who was looking for subjects to enrol in a multi-centred, randomized, controlled clinical trial sponsored by the Alzheimer's Society. Dr. Selleck was one of three investigators. The trial was intended to test a new drug, Tetrahydroaminoacridine (THA), which promises to reduce dramatically the progression rate of Alzheimer's disease.

Owing to the nature of THA and the mechanisms by which it works, the investigators wanted subjects who were more or less in the middle stages of Alzheimer's, where serious impairment of mental function is in evidence but not to the point where the subject has lost complete control of all mental capacities. Patients at this stage of the disease tend to experience "intermittent competency." Given the size of the population at St. Mary's, Dr. Selleck figured that there must be a substantial number of elderly patients who met the criteria for inclusion in the study.

After explaining the nature of the proposed study, Dr. Selleck asked Ann Wilson for permission to visit St. Mary's to interview and recruit potential research subjects. She indicated that she would enrol a patient in the study only if: (a) the patient provided formal, written consent; (b) the patient's closest relative provided formal, written consent; and (c) no one on the health-care staff at St. Mary's, including Ann Wilson, had any objection to including the patient in the study. If the patient has been ruled "legally incompetent," then condition (a) would be ignored and formal consent would be sought only from the nearest relative. If, for any patient, including those who were intermittently competent, there was no relative available, then that patient would be excluded from consideration altogether.

After hearing Dr. Selleck's proposal, Ann Wilson made the following reply. "Why don't I save us all a lot of time and bother? I simply will not permit elderly patients under my care to be used as guinea pigs in a clinical trial. These are extremely vulnerable people we're talking about here, not people in their prime. They've been through enough in their lives already without being subject to scientific examination, or should I say 'exploitation.' The elderly population, especially those who are institutionalized and suffering from serious impairment of mental function, are a vulnerable group who should not be used in medical experiments, even for 'noble' purposes. I just won't allow it – not in my nursing home!"

Dr. Selleck expressed considerable surprise at this response. She indicated that without access to St. Mary's, it would be virtually impossible for her to make the appropriate contact with the elderly residents and their families. And without a significant number of recruits from St. Mary's, her sample size would not be large enough, scientifically, for her to participate in the multi-centred trial. She indicated further that the proposed trial had been examined by her Hospital's Research Ethics Board, who had given it their whole-hearted endorsement. It had also been approved by the Research Ethics Boards from which her other two investigators were required to receive approval. Despite these appeals, Ann Wilson would not budge. "Not in my nursing home," she repeated.

Was Ann Wilson right to object to Dr. Selleck's proposed clinical trial?

Case Discussion

(1) Institutionalization

One crucial issue in the Wilson case arises from the not insubstantial difference between, on the one hand, the elderly person living at home, in an environment in which she has autonomy and control and a consequent sense of dignity and self-worth; and on the other, the person living in an institutional environment over which she has comparatively little control and in which she is dependent upon others. She is, as Kantians and feminist ethicists would put it, subject to the will of others. As Warren Reich notes,

> a significant ethical issue arises in the context of research among elderly persons in nursing homes, homes for the aged, geriatric wards, and institutions for the mentally infirm, insofar as they are captive populations subject to exploitation in general and a diminution of freedom and voluntariness in particular.[1]

He adds that,

Whether or not the residents of those institutions are intellectually competent, the demeaning treatment, the dependence created by institutionalization, and the powerful inducement to conform to institutional expectations create inherent coercions, constraints, and obstacles to both competent and free (voluntary) consent in a significant number of these institutions.[2]

We do not have to conjure up horror stories concerning physical and emotional abuse of institutionalized patients to appreciate this point; we needn't indulge in "institution bashing." In the warmest and most caring of institutional settings – perhaps in these settings more than others! – pressures to conform, to contribute, and to please those upon whom one is dependent may be latent and very powerful. These may render the choice to engage in a research project less than fully voluntary.

This is true, of course, of any person in any institutional setting, be it a prison, a hospital, or even a university. But the pressures may be even stronger in the case of institutionalized, elderly persons, owing to their traditional positions within our society. Many elderly persons conceive of themselves as relatively unproductive and unnecessary compared with younger people. Some also conceive of themselves as burdens upon society, in particular those members of society upon whom they are in some way dependent, such as a spouse, a child, a relative, or a professional care-provider. One sometimes hears claims like, "As soon as I hit sixty-five I was suddenly no longer useful to anyone." And even if elderly persons don't perceive themselves in this way, there appear to be many others who do. One also sometimes hears comments like, "Don't worry yourself about that; let me take care of things for you." Or, "Let me worry about that. At this stage in your life you deserve to put your feet up and take things easy." Well-intentioned as they might be, and there is little doubt that for the most part they are, such comments, and the actions which accompany them, betray a conception of elderly people as helpless, non-contributing, no-longer-vital and possibly burdensome members of society.

Given this conception, and the self-perceptions which it cannot help but foster, a researcher may well find herself in a potentially exploitive position – a position to exploit, intentionally or unwittingly, the vulnerability of elderly persons. Many elderly people will be especially keen for the opportunity to contribute to society through participation in important research studies. Yet as Reich notes, "the elderly should not be made victims of their own altruism or of the *need to be needed*."[3] One can imagine the force that this need must have in the case of elderly people, especially those who are institutionally dependent, though the need must be evident in other cases as well. One can imagine the feeling of one who, for most of a lifetime, has thought of herself as, and has been thought by others to be, an essential, contributing member of society, but who now finds herself no longer viewed in this way. Instead she is viewed much as a helpless infant. How tempting it must be, readily and perhaps without due care and consideration of her own interests, to accede to a request to contribute to "valuable" medical research, thereby asserting once again her value, worth, and autonomy.

The above having been noted, however, the question arises whether the proper way of protecting institutionalized elderly people from this kind of vulnerability is to deny them the opportunity to involve themselves in research projects. In the present case the question is whether there are ways of protecting the patients of St. Mary's from potential exploitation which are less offensive than the course pursued by Ann Wilson. Was she being unduly paternalistic? Was she unjustifiably treating her patients as helpless infants? Was her protectionist policy in violation of Kant's categorical imperative to respect the rational autonomy of other people? Could a rule prohibiting all research on the institutionalized elderly find its way into a moral code which maximized utility over the long run?

We will return to these questions later.

(2) Intermittent Competency

Another key issue in some cases involving the elderly arises from the phenomenon of intermittent and partial competency. In law, and the thinking of many people, each adult person is presumed to be competent unless proven otherwise. In addition, competency is generally viewed as a strictly all-or-nothing affair. That is, in law adults are presumed to be fully competent, and if that presumption is to be defeated, the only alternative is that the person in question is fully incompetent. There is no in-between, no room for degrees of competency. Yet mental competency does appear to come in degrees and may fluctuate over time. In the case of the elderly, one sometimes encounters the "sunshine phenomenon," the tendency to display lucidity, alertness, and other cognitive capacities to a comparatively greater degree first thing in the day and to increasingly lesser degrees as the day progresses.

Given these facts about elderly persons (indeed about persons in general), one should be wary of employing, consciously or otherwise, the legal model in selecting subjects for experimental research. It would be a mistake to infer that because an elderly person has not been shown to be fully incompetent she is therefore fully competent, and to conclude from this that one therefore need not worry at all about the capacity for informed consent. If there are many points lying between full competence and full incompetence, and if a person just might occupy different points at different times, then any such inferences would be invalid and fraught with danger. One would, in drawing such a conclusion, be sweeping under the rug the hard choices that must be made, and simply ignoring potentially disastrous effects. There is, of course, great temptation to do this. It is far more difficult to establish degrees or grades of competency than it is to establish outright incompetence. It may be even more difficult to determine where along the spectrum lying between the two extremes one should begin to draw lines, where one should begin to question whether consent is truly informed, voluntary, and therefore valid.

It may be a virtue of Dr. Selleck's research protocol that an attempt was to be made to secure consent both from the elderly patients and from their families. Such a move may serve to protect the patient's interests when an erroneous judgment of competence is made. But now ask the following question: if consent of both parties is required, and if a reasonably competent patient consents but the family member does not, does it not seriously violate the autonomy of the patient to bar her from the study? Does this not subject one individual to the will of another? Maybe so. But then the question becomes which is more urgent to protect: the right of a patient, falsely judged to be competent, to the protection afforded by the requirement of family consent, or the autonomy-right of the competent patient who is in disagreement with his relative? The question becomes even more complicated, of course, given the role assigned to Ann Wilson and her staff. Should they have what is in effect a veto over patient participation? It is one thing to seek the informed opinion of professionals entrusted with a patient's care, quite another to allow them effectively to make a negative decision for the patient. Perhaps the rights of the St. Mary's residents are being violated by both Ann Wilson and Dr. Selleck!

(3) Special Class?

The considerations discussed in the preceding two sections may suggest that the elderly constitute a special class of persons deserving of special consideration and protection. It may be that legislators, Ethics Review Boards, medical researchers, and the heads of nursing homes for the elderly should designate or consider the elderly, along with children, human embryos, and the irreversibly comatose, a special class for whom special rules are appropriate. And perhaps those rules should exclude the elderly from consideration for medical research altogether, as Ann Wilson apparently thought.

Despite the apparent attractiveness of these conclusions, some serious reservations may be expressed about accepting them. First, it is misleading to speak simply in terms of elderly persons, or even elderly patients. The differences in the situations of elderly people seem far too numerous and important for us to do that. For instance, one might ponder the important differences represented in the following six scenarios.

1. First, there is the elderly couple living at home, both fully competent, in control of their affairs and experiencing considerable satisfaction in life.
2. Then there is the elderly person living at home with his spouse upon whom he is, to some degree anyway, dependent for emotional and physical needs. Perhaps he is in the middle stages of Alzheimer's.
3. There is also the elderly person living at home with a person other than his spouse, perhaps with a relative, friend or professional care-giver. This person is physically dependent but in no way mentally or emotionally impaired and dependent.
4. Consider this same person living in a nursing home, or some other facility in which professional care is provided.
5. A fifth case concerns an elderly person living in such a facility whose mental competence is only intermittent or partial.
6. Finally, we might consider an elderly person living in such a facil-

ity who is suffering from severe senile dementia and whose mental incompetence is unquestionable.

The above six scenarios are by no means exhaustive, but they do raise an important question which needs to be asked. Is it morally dangerous to speak of "the elderly" as a distinct class? Are the differences in the situations of elderly people far too numerous to allow such a classification to be useful? Will different scenarios involving different elderly people raise crucially different moral questions concerning the involvement of elderly people in medical research? Consider how one might respond if the class in question were not the elderly but, say, women. Any attempt to categorize along the lines of gender would be highly objectionable. There are far too many relevant differences among women, for purposes of medical research studies, to make this a useful and non-offensive category upon which to base the right to consent to participation in medical research studies. Use of any such category would be considered highly discriminatory. Might the same not be said of age?

A second, related worry is that by pursuing the "protected class" option, legitimate concern could well develop into concern of a rather unfortunate kind. It might develop into a full-fledged paternalism which would wreak far more damage than it could ever prevent. As Richard Ratzan puts it,

> The most insidious loss of liberty for an elderly subject, *and the one least likely to be detected and corrected* is paternalism. The elderly often do need help in providing for themselves and thereby set the stage for what Lionel Trilling called the dangers which lie in our most generous wishes ... to go on to make [our fellow human beings] the objects of our *pity*, then of our *wisdom*, ultimately of our *coercion*.[4]

There are many possible effects of paternalism in the case of the elderly. First, there is the possibility of genuine harm to the subject. Paternalism could lead to an underestimation of the capacities of the elderly to exercise as much enlightened freedom of decision as any "ordinary person" concerning what might or might not be harmful to them. This in turn might lead a researcher, or a guardian, unnecessarily and unjustifiably to substitute his less enlightened judgment. It might also lead the researcher sometimes to withhold possibly disturbing information from the potential research subject. Recall the line noted earlier: "Don't worry yourself about that; let me take care of things for you." All this can lead to significant harm in addition to loss of liberty and autonomy, a harm which must not be underestimated (as Kant so rightly pointed out). What may appear, through the eyes of a healthy 30-year-old, as an inconsequential inconvenience or physical discomfort might be experienced as a serious physical harm by an elderly person. Harm, as with beauty and its beholder, lies to some degree in the eyes of its victim.

A second possible effect of the paternalism implicit in the protected class option lies in what Ratzan terms "the revocation of what many elderly subjects desire and feel is their right to volunteer, to help others, to participate."[5] It is wise to be wary of tendencies to exaggerate problems such as vulnerability and lack of competency. It is also wise to be sceptical of attempts to seek, as a corrective to such problems, measures which err in the opposite direction. Disqualifying potential subjects who really are, so long as reasonable precautions are taken to avoid exploitation, quite able rationally to make up their own minds – to disqualify them, in the end, mainly because of their age – smacks of a form of discrimination we might call "ageism."

A third possible effect of the protected class option is that exaggerated concern for the elderly patient might lead to a blanket prohibition on all research involving all elderly people. Yet as Neil Chayet puts it in relation to similar movements to bar all research involving mentally incompetent elderly persons, "if prohibition of research continues to be the protective device that is utilized, we may well 'protect' thousands of persons to death or to lives of misery."[6] If the only viable way of testing new procedures to help future elderly, but incompetent, persons suffering from afflictions like Alzheimer's is to do research using those presently afflicted, then how will medical science progress if we bar all such research? The same question arises in the present case, although here the possibility exists for valid, informed consent so long as we are careful.

Ageism is a form of discrimination into which it is very easy to fall. This is largely explained, no doubt, by one simple fact. Paternalistically based ageism, though discriminatory, is almost always motivated by a worthy aim: the good of another person. This distinguishes ageism from most other forms of discrimination which are usually motivated by ignoble aims such as hatred, ignorance, or the desire to oppress another racial or religious group. Given this important difference, it is quite easy for the "ageist" to distance himself from the usual forms of discrimination, to deny or not even notice that what he is doing bears a significant resemblance to racism and sexism. After all, the ageist will ask, how can it be wrong to be concerned with the good of another person? Yet this can be wrong if the concern amounts to over-concern – and one must be especially vigilant of this possibility when dealing with the elderly, especially those dependent upon institutional care.

(5) Treatment as an Individual

The dangers of ageism may make one hesitant even to speak or conceive of the elderly, including the institutionalized elderly, as a special group. One may be especially hesitant in suggesting separate and distinct protections over and above the protections afforded all individuals by the ethical requirements of research on human subjects. Perhaps we would do well to heed the advice of those who claim that "there is no special need to regard the aged as a distinct class in terms of the requirements of research guidelines: some of the aged are competent, others are not."[7] If this is correct, then it would be wrong to conceive of age as itself a morally relevant consideration, as Ann Wilson may have done. To be sure, age often brings with it such difficulties as incompetency, institutional dependency, and vulnerability, and researchers should be aware of this fact. But perhaps we are better off, for purposes of research, if we talk in terms of these difficulties and not age itself. We are better off if we treat the elderly as *individual persons*, some, but not all, of whom suffer these difficulties than if we conceive of them as constituting a group – the aged – for whom special protection is required. Such a conception, coupled with natural, paternalistic inclinations, could lead to morally undesirable consequences.

Perhaps the same is true whether we are talking of the elderly, the institutionalized elderly, or even elderly persons suffering from diseases like Alzheimer's, or from partial or intermittent competency. If so, then one must question the propriety of the blanket restriction proposed by Ann Wilson. On the other hand, if the potential harms of paternalism and ageism are worth risking for the sake of protecting those who might falsely be judged competent and allowed to consent, then perhaps she is right after all. Perhaps she is right in saying: "Not in my nursing home!"

Notes

1   Warren T. Reich, "Ethical Issues Related to Research Involving Elderly Subjects," *The Gerontologist,* August, 1978, 18(4), 333.
2   Reich.
3   Reich, 331.
4   Richard Ratzan, "'Being Old Makes You Different': The Elderly as Research Subjects," *Hastings Center Reports*, Vol. 10, no. 5 (1980), 36.
5   Ratzan.
6   Ratzan.
7   Reich, 326.

Chapter 6: Mental Illness

Case 6:1 Non-Consensual Electro-Convulsive Shock Therapy

Mr. S. is a 53-year-old widowed father of one child. He was brought by ambulance to the Emergency Department of Toronto's Hospital X after a neighbour found him unconscious on the bed. There was an empty bottle of Elavil, an anti-depressant, on the night table. After 36 hours in the Intensive Care Unit, he was transferred to the in-patient Psychiatry Unit at Hospital Y.

On admission Mr. S. was agitated, restless, and paced up and down the ward almost incessantly. He was haggard and tearful most of the time. Mr. S. reported difficulty in concentrating and remembering things and felt his brain was "rotting." He showed little interest in ward activities and was reluctant to talk to the staff or to other patients. Over the next few days it was noted he was neglecting his appearance. He was unshaven, unkempt, and his clothes were put on carelessly. He woke up most mornings at 4 or 4:30 and was unable to go back to sleep.

Although his son reported that his father was relatively well-off, Mr. S. claimed repeatedly that he was on the verge of financial ruin and in danger of losing the family home. He also felt extremely guilty about not being at home when his mother had died thirty-two years before, and kept repeating that if only he had been there she would not have died. The future appeared bleak, with no hope that it would get better. He kept repeating that living in a state of perpetual depression was intolerable and he would rather be dead than suffer like this for the rest of his life.

On the third evening after Mr. S.'s admission to the Psychiatric Unit the nurse found him fashioning a noose out of his pillowcase. He admitted that he was going to sneak into the bathroom with it and hang himself from one of the fixtures. If that failed, he vowed he would try to electrocute himself or find a way to get sufficient pills for an overdose.

The psychiatrist proposed a course of six electroconvulsive shock treatments (ECT) over a two-week period. Mr. S. refused to consent to the proposed treatment. He insisted that he had no desire to live, that indeed there was nothing to live for in his present state, and pleaded with the psychiatrist just to be left alone. After all it was his life. Why were the doctors and nurses so bent on preventing him from taking his life?

When Mr. S.'s son was invited to sign the consent form on his father's behalf, he refused to override his father's expressed wishes. Furthermore, he had heard all sorts of bad things about ECT: stories of vertebral fractures, permanent memory loss, heart failure, and even death. He just could not bring himself to expose his father to such risks. Instead he requested the continuation of drug therapy because he perceived this to be a less invasive and safer form of treatment.

On hearing the son's worries about the effects of the treatment, the psychiatrist tried to reassure him that the memory loss sustained was temporary, and that while cardiac arrhythmias are not uncommon following the stimulus, these usually subside without after-effects. Furthermore, he assured the son that, while the mortality rates in the early days of ECT were significant, the present mortality rates were very low.

On the son's proposal to continue drug therapy, the psychiatrist pointed out that the initial treatment with anti-depressant drugs had neither reduced his father's severe depression nor prevented him from attempting to take his life. For psychotic depression the best short-term results were likely to be achieved by ECT. In cases similar to his father's, ECT had dramatically addressed the severe depression, reduced the threat of suicide, and enabled patients to function well with maintenance-drug therapy. Would a more invasive form of therapy not be preferable if it stood a better chance of preventing the possibility of a further suicide attempt?

Despite all attempts to overcome young Mr. S.'s fears, he remained adamant and refused to sign the consent form, insisting that he should respect his father's refusal of treatment. After all, even though his father was depressed he was not mentally incompetent.

In view of this stalemate, should the psychiatrist apply to Ontario's Review Board for permission to treat Mr. S. with ECT against his wishes and those of his son?[1]

Case Discussion

(1) ECT: The Procedure

As a medical procedure electroconvulsive treatment has been employed for over forty years. During that time it has proved to be effective in the treatment of severe depression. As is the case with so many of our medical interventions, however, it is not known why ECT works.

The procedure involves running a charge of electricity through the brain. This may be done unilaterally or bilaterally. The unilateral technique involves placing one electrode over the non-dominant hemisphere of the brain. By contrast, the bilateral technique requires that the electrodes be placed on both temples in order to expose both hemispheres to the electrical current.

A single shock uses about the same amount of energy as a 100 watt electric bulb. This charge of electricity induces a convulsive seizure. For reasons unknown, this procedure offers symptomatic relief from severe depression. A single treatment, from start to finish, takes about three to five minutes. A typical series for depression is six to twelve separate shocks, administered at two to three day intervals. Short term memory loss invariably follows treatment. In a small number of cases the memory loss can be long-term or permanent. There is also some dispute as to whether or not long time use of ECT causes brain damage (as revealed in autopsies).[2]

Popular fears about ECT have probably been intensified by media depictions as in the movie *One Flew Over the Cuckoo's Nest*. Nowadays patients are partially anaesthetized to eliminate pain. Muscle relaxants are administered to prevent violent contortions and bone fractures. Oxygen is also administered, since muscles controlling breathing are paralysed during the procedure.

(2) Is ECT Medically Indicated in This Case?

(a) **Diagnosis**
Mr. S. exhibits the tell-tale marks of severe depression with psychotic features. He is tearful, haggard, shows little interest in what goes on around him, is neglectful of his appearance, and sleeps poorly. Furthermore, he appears to be "out of touch with reality"; witness his

fears about his financial straits and his assessment of the events surrounding his mother's death.

(b) Efficacy of ECT in Severe Depression

Published controlled studies of ECT confirm its short-term efficacy in cases of severe depression. Some studies rate it equally efficacious as, and others superior to, drug therapy.[3] "Not a single controlled study has shown another form of treatment to be superior to ECT in the short-term management of depression."[4] Preference for ECT where there is an immediate risk of suicide is related to the fact that it works much faster. In the present case the whole series of treatments would be over by the time drugs would begin to take effect (on average in four to six weeks).

(3) Competence and Consent To Treatment

Contrary to popular beliefs about mentally-ill patients, "the overwhelming majority of such patients are quite competent to give valid consent."[5] Does Mr. S. fall into this category of mentally-ill but not necessarily mentally incompetent patients? If he does then on what grounds, if any, may his wishes and those of his son be bypassed?

(4) Health-care Professionals' Perspective

(a) Promising Prognosis

By training and perhaps by temperament, health-care professionals are predisposed to save lives and ameliorate suffering. The present case provides an opportunity for doing both. ECT might well eliminate Mr. S.'s suicidal tendencies and dramatically reduce, even though not entirely eradicate, his severe depression. Acknowledgement of these probable boons should not blind us, however, to the limitations of ECT. It is well known that the procedure is efficacious only in the short term and that in the first year following its use the relapse rates are likely to be high unless maintenance antidepressant medications are subsequently prescribed. Because this is known, it is extremely unlikely that Mr. S. would be subjected to electro-convulsive shock treatment without maintenance-drug therapy. In combination the two treatment forms hold promise of improved mental health.

(b) The Principle of Utility

In this case it is difficult to dodge the question of whether the patient's expressed wishes may be ignored in favour of promoting his best interests. Would an appeal to the principle of utility justify acting paternalistically for the patient's own good? Would this depend on whether the principle applied to the actions contemplated in this case, or to a general rule to be followed in all similar cases? Whatever the answer, the appeals to utility work most effectively when comparing patients' states (of suffering) at one time with those at another time. In the present case this would involve comparing Mr. S.'s severe depression now with probably less severe depression later. Doubtless Mr. S. could conceivably offer a different comparison – severe depression now versus no depression later. If he is left to his own devices suicide will take care of his depression. Unfortunately, this drastic measure "cures" the "disease" by killing the patient. Because the principle of utility is geared to comparing lesser with greater states of suffering (or happiness), not severe states of suffering with non-existence, it fails, strictly speaking, to apply in this kind of case. Comparisons of states of suffering are predicated on the continued existence of the patient.

Even if one looks on the bleak side and the envisaged favourable prognosis turns out to be incorrect, should that retrospective wisdom furnish an occasion for regret? Suppose that, instead of improving after treatment, Mr. S.'s depression persists and he succeeds in committing suicide. Should the members of the treatment team wish they had not intervened? They saved him yesterday only to lose him today. To be sure, that would be an occasion for regret. But one needs accurately to pinpoint the cause of it. Should we regret having administered the most effective known treatment for Mr. S.'s depression, or regret that the most effective treatment available proved to be inadequate? Would that retrospective wisdom absolve them from the responsibility of treating another severely depressed patient tomorrow with Mr. S.'s prospects of benefit? When, in the semi-darkness of ignorance of outcome, we are faced with the decision to treat mentally-ill patients like Mr. S., can we be sure that their refusals of treatment are infallible indicators that they find the prospect of death preferable to life? Or is this their depression speaking? When in doubt about treating such patients, it could be argued that the doubt should be resolved in favour of life.

(c) **Promoting versus Expressing Autonomy**

Patient autonomy or the right to self-determination is closely related to respect for the patient as a person. Such respect has emerged in the evolution of the physician-patient relationship from a paternalistic to a more collegial model. Lacking proportionate reasons one may not override the patient's expressed wishes. If, in the present case, the treatment team are given the "green light" to treat Mr. S. against his wishes, those ministrations could hardly be designated as expressive of his autonomy. It takes little imagination, however, to see that while subjecting a patient to ECT against his expressed wishes now is not expressive of patient autonomy, it may contribute to the restoration and/or enlargement of that autonomy later. If treatment relieves Mr. S.'s depression, at a later point in time it will in all likelihood expand his ability to function. Do health-care professionals have any obligation to aid and abet patient behaviour that is momentarily expressive of self-determination, but which is causally ineffective in producing it in the long run (given that the patient will likely kill himself?

(5) Patient's Perspective

(a) **Limits of Paternalism**

This case also raises the question of whether we may interfere with or constrain others when their actions are likely to harm only themselves and not others. This is not to deny that Mr. S. may not harm others in the sense that others, particularly members of his family and close friends, would grieve and be distressed should he succeed in a future attempt to commit suicide. It is moot, however, whether patients have an obligation to endure severe and prolonged suffering to spare friends and loved ones the grief of bereavement. A similar argument may be advanced against members of the treatment team who experience difficulties with patients' refusal of treatment. Should patients undergoing unbearable or unacceptable suffering be kept alive against their wishes as a means of minimizing uncomfortable feelings in health-care givers?

The main fear that needs to be addressed in this business about mentally-ill patients harming themselves rather than harming others stems from uncertainty. How can we be sure that Mr. S. may not become assaultive? Can we be certain that "apparently harmless" mentally-ill patients won't become aggressive and injure others around them? The answer is, "Of course we can't." But if one is prepared to gear one's responses to probabilities rather than remote possibilities the fear that Mr. S., if untreated, may become violent appears to be groundless. At no point in the history of the treatment of Mr. S. has he exhibited behaviour that may be characterized as "dangerous." To allow violation of his autonomy on grounds of a remote possibility that might later prove dangerous, when we would clearly *not* licence such a denial in the case of a person who is not mentally ill, would be to discriminate against Mr. S. on grounds of mental illness.

(b) On the Right to Change One's Mind

Earlier Mr. S. had submitted to drug therapy. Should we take his prior acceptance of treatment as expressive of his genuine wishes rather than his present refusal, in a severely depressed state, of a potentially life-saving measure? But wasn't Mr. S. in a depressed state when he consented earlier to treatment? Perhaps his present refusal of treatment is related to his disappointment with the lack of improvement in his condition in spite of his previous acquiescence. Are we to understand his initial acquiescence as an irrevocable commitment to treatment? If so, why do we view things differently in the case of the cancer patient who initially agrees to surgery but who now refuses chemotherapy? How can we acknowledge the right of patients to refuse potentially life-saving treatment in the one case but not in the other? Is this not, once again, discriminatory?

(c) Sovereignty Over One's Own Life

According to Schopenhauer, "it is quite obvious that there is nothing in the world to which every man has a more unassailable title than to his own life and person." Why do physicians sometimes value patients' lives more than the patients themselves? This may be attributed, at least in part, to the fact that health-care professionals frequently perceive death as a failure. This outlook may then find expression in a form of medical vitalism that results "in extolling mental health and physical survival over every other value, particularly individual liberty."[6] Earlier we challenged the application of the principle of utility to this present case, pointing out that, strictly speaking, the principle may not be applicable. However, that is not the last word on the subject. May there not be states of life worse than death? May not quality of life be so poor, or be perceived to be so poor, that death may be rationally deemed preferable? If not, on whose value scale is the decision to be based? The patient's, the family's, or the health care professionals'? Must patient preferences for death to life in a state of severe suffering or pain be taken as infallible indicators of mental incompetence? The crucial question at stake in this case is whether we are justified in drawing as sharp a distinction between physical and mental illness as we do, especially when we feel confident that we may be dealing with valid but unreasonable refusal of treatment rather than mental incompetence.

(d) The Right to Treat: Claim-Right or Privilege?

In the current literature in biomedical ethics much is made of the right to refuse treatment. Paul Ramsey insists that the right to refuse treatment is a relative rather than an absolute right. There are "medically indicated treatments...that a competent conscious patient has no moral right to refuse, just as one has no moral right to deliberately ruin his life."[7] To argue otherwise would "reduce medical ethics to patient autonomy ..."[8] and turn physicians into "animated tools" (Aristotle's label for a slave). While Ramsey may be essentially correct in claiming that the right to refuse treatment is a relative right, it is a short step from the position he advocates to a confusion of the physician's privilege to treat a patient with a claim right. Consent to a medical treatment grants a privilege to the physician to intervene. Ramsey comes close to translating a "privilege" into a "claim right" which imposes a correlative obligation on the patient to submit to treatment – a move which, if it were permitted, would make a travesty of consent. With this in mind, consider now the practice of skewing the physician-patient relationship in favour of paternalism rather than patient autonomy. Can we consistently universalize treating patients against their wishes even when it is "for their own good"? If not, may we avoid reducing medical ethics to patient autonomy by introducing a bona fide exception of the form, "The patient's right to refuse treatment must be respected except when the patient is likely to commit suicide if not treated"? Or is the patient's right to self-determination paramount even in the context of the threat of suicide?

Notes

1   The relevance of this question is unaffected by amendments to the *Mental Health Act of Ontario* [Attorney General's Equality of Rights Status law Amendment Act, 1986 (Bill 7)]. Section 35(4)(a),

which came into force April 1, 1987, empowers Review Boards to issue an order to treat an involuntary psychiatric patient even when the patient is mentally competent to refuse treatment.

2   George H. Kieffer, *Bioethics* (Reading, MA: Addison-Wesley, 1979), 269.

3   "Electro-Convulsive Therapy," U.S. Consensus Development Conference Statement, vol. 5, No.11.

4   "Electro-Convulsive Therapy."

5   Charles M. Culver and Bernard Gert, *Philosophy in Medicine* (New York: Oxford University Press, 1982), 61.

6   Thomas Szasz, *Primary Values and Major Contentions* (Amherst, NJ: Prometheus, 1983), 36.

7   Paul Ramsey, *Ethics at the Edges of Life* (Hew Haven, CT: Yale University Press. 1978), 156.

8   Ramsey.

Case 6:2 Discontinuing Forced Feeding of an Anorexia Nervosa Patient

Amelda is a 21-year-old, unmarried, female patient suffering from anorexia nervosa. Her parents emigrated to Canada from the Philippines when she was a baby. Amelda's father is a successful businessman belonging to the upper-middle class. The other members of the family are Amelda's older brother and two younger sisters. Members of the family are practising Roman Catholics. The family may be accurately described as "western" in outlook.

During the past three years Amelda has been admitted fifteen times to the psychiatric unit at Fairweather Hospital. A wide range of treatment regimens have been employed, including individual psychotherapy, family therapy, antidepressant and antipsychotic drugs, electroconvulsive therapy, and behaviour modification.

All attempts at treatment so far have failed. All efforts at feeding have been frustrated by Amelda's self-destructive behaviour. She has refused solid foods, repeatedly removed her naso-gastric tube, withdrawn nutritional supplements from her stomach with a syringe, and over-dosed herself with laxatives. The only successful deterrent to this behaviour has been physical restraints. Even physical restraints, however, have not prevented her from doing isometric exercises that have successfully reduced her weight.

Amelda exudes an air of sadness and describes herself as being depressed most of the time. Despite her thin, emaciated appearance – she weighs 36.5 kg (80.7 lb) – she perceives herself as obese and is revolted by food and the sounds of mastication and swallowing.

Although her higher cognitive functions are normal, Amelda's insight and judgment are poor. She objects to force-feeding. While she has expressed no desire to die, she does not believe that she needs as much food as her physicians claim in order to live. Isn't the fact that she is still alive despite all their warnings proof of this?

Physicians, other health-care professionals, and members of Amelda's family have reached an impasse and are now querying the wisdom of continuing to force-feed her. To stop force-feeding, however, would probably result in death. Amelda's past medical history confirms that whenever her weight falls below 35 kg (77 lb) her blood pressure, electrolytes, and haemoglobin drop to dangerously low levels, threatening her life. If allowed to continue to lose weight, Amelda is likely to become confused, then comatose, or she would develop a cardiac arrhythmia and die. The question then to be faced is whether she should be resuscitated if she were to suffer cardiac arrest.

Would health-care professionals, with the agreement of Amelda's family, be morally justified in refraining from force-feeding her, and, in the event of cardiac arrest resisting resuscitative measures?

Case Discussion

(1) Clinical Criteria

Amelda exhibits the classic symptoms of anorexia nervosa. These are: (a) intense fear of becoming obese, which does not diminish as weight loss progresses; (b) disturbance of body image, i.e., claiming to "feel fat" even when emaciated; (c) weight loss of at least 25 per cent of original body weight; (d) refusal to maintain body weight over a minimal weight for age and height; and (e) no known physical illness that would account for the weight loss.[1]

What of Amelda's depression? The relationship between anorexia nervosa and depression is complex. When self-esteem is intimately linked to weight and appearance, perception of oneself as obese may contribute to self-loathing and depression. Depression may also be a physiological effect of starvation.[2]

(2) Treatment So Far

The whole gamut of available therapies has been run in Amelda's case, to no avail. These include: (a) individual psychotherapy aimed at helping the patient to regain physical health, reduce symptoms, increase self-esteem, and make progress in personal and social development; (b) family therapy intended to establish appropriate eating patterns, to facilitate communication, and to permit family members to relate better to one another; (c) antidepressant drugs and ECT for relief of depression; (d) antipsychotic drugs, which serve a dual purpose. They have a sedative function, aimed at controlling agitation and overexercising, and they also stimulate appetite; (e) behaviour modification designed to encourage patient compliance with treatment regimen through a system of rewards.

(3) Possible Reasons for Discontinuing Force-Feeding

(a) Until the various options to treat have been tried and proved to be unsuccessful, the health-care team had a mandate to force-feed Amelda. Now that all attempts to cure or ameliorate her condition have failed, that mandate has run out.

(b) Since Amelda objects to force-feeding, the decision to terminate it would not violate her autonomy.

(c) Since she is not being actively treated for her illness, mere preservation of life is not a sufficient warrant for keeping her in an acute care ward.

(d) While stopping force-feeding is life threatening, death is not inevitable. Entrusting her with the life-death decision may jolt her into assuming responsibility for her own life.

(4) Obstacles to Terminating Force-Feeding

(a) Termination of force-feeding once it has continued for as long as four years is difficult, at least psychologically, even if the foregoing reasons are basically sound. Recall Aristotle's claim that moral acts spring from settled dispositions which we call virtues. It "goes against the grain" for individuals who exhibit the virtues of benevolence and compassion to contemplate not feeding a vulnerable patient who requires nourishment to live.

(b) Failure to feed a patient is perceived to be morally blameworthy in a way that withholding other forms of treatment is not. This is evident in the furore over the recent decision of the Council on Ethical and Judicial Affairs of the American Medical Association that it is not unethical to withhold food and water and other amenities from patients in an irreversible coma. Philosopher Patrick Derr objects, "Deciding to begin selective starvation is a decision no civilization should make."[3] Concerns were also raised about the slippery slope toward wholesale euthanasia (see Case 8:3). If objections to withholding feeding from irreversible comatose patients are so strong, they are likely to be even stronger in the present case.

(c) Force-feeding (i.e., one form of treating a patient against her expressed wishes) is justifiable when the patient is mentally incompetent. Amelda was certified to be incompetent on each of her admissions to hospital. Issues surrounding surrogate consent now enter the picture (see Case 5:1).

(d) While, as noted earlier, force-feeding was undertaken initially with a view to curing or ameliorating the patient's condition, this cannot have been true latterly. For some time certification and force-feeding were adopted as the means to preserve Amelda's life. On the basis of the sanctity-of-life principle, it could be argued that without life there would be no hope of improving the quality of Amelda's life. Hence force-feeding is justified if it preserves her life.

(e) If it is argued that quality of life should enter into the reckoning, two questions then arise: (i) Who judges that quality of life has diminished to the point where it should no longer be sustained? and (ii) On the basis of what criteria is that judgment made? Amelda obviously finds life tolerable on the terms she has "elected" to live it. Once again, issues involving surrogate consent enter the picture.

(f) Rather than terminate force-feeding, with its attendant risk of death, would it not be preferable to try to get Amelda admitted to a chronic care facility, thus undercutting the cost/benefit objection to maintaining her in an acute care ward?

(5) Exploring the Do-Not-Resuscitate Option

The case for discontinuing force-feeding is coupled with a query about the appropriateness of writing a DNR (Do-Not-Resuscitate) order. The two proposals certainly give every appearance of compatibility. Indeed, what reason could we possibly give for refusing to write a DNR order once the decision to discontinue force-feeding has been made? Is there not an inconsistency in advocating that force-feeding be discontinued, but then stopping short of writing a DNR order? We decide to terminate force-feeding knowing that Amelda may suffer cardiac arrest, but when she does we resuscitate. Why? So that we can refuse to force-feed her again and have her arrest so we can resuscitate once more? In Kantian terms, would such a regimen, if expressed in a moral rule, not yield a self-contradictory maxim, a maxim that would fail to pass the test of the Categorical Imperative?

Consider too, whether this inconsistency infects Amelda's own thinking. She opposes force-feeding and this opposition places her at risk of lowering her bodily resistance and rendering her vulnerable, among other things, to cardiac arrest. But she has not expressed the wish to die. For whatever reason, she does not seem to be able to grasp that refusal of force-feeding is causally linked, not to one, but to two outcomes: (i) maintenance of low weight-level (which she finds desirable), and (ii) risk of death (which she does not take seriously). Up to the present she has been able to get (i) without (ii), but at the expense of the concern expressed in 3 (c) above – an irresponsible, non-cost-effective utilization of scarce medical resources in an acute care hospital. The question arises: Is it appropriate for physicians and health-care professionals to think like policy-makers at the bedside, or should they simply utilize all possible resources for the benefit of their patients, with no questions asked? The term "benefit" is ambiguous here. Under the present regimen, benefit amounts to preserving Amelda's life. All attempts at restoring her to more "normal" levels of functioning have failed. Concerns about a wise use of resources focus on that very failure to enhance Amelda's quality of life. Is there any way that the claims of life and quality of life can be harmonized in this case?

(6) Legal Considerations

The following observations emerged in consultation with a lawyer about the possible legal repercussions of discontinuing force-feeding, and about the advisability of coupling that proposal with the writing of a DNR order.

(a) Legal Roadblocks to the Discontinuation of Force-Feeding
(i) The patient's right to refuse treatment, with the exception of mentally incompetent patients, is recognized in Canadian and American law. Since Amelda has been consistently certified as mentally incompetent on each of her previous admissions, her right to refuse treatment is nullified and health-care professionals have the privilege, indeed the duty, to provide her with protection and care.
(ii) Treatment, once initiated, and in this case continued for a period of four years, may not be withdrawn without adequate justification.
(iii) During the session with the lawyer, it was proposed that Amelda be decertified, thus paving the way for acquiescence in her wishes not to be force fed. The lawyer pointed out that this would be inconsistent with the practice of the past four years. In this

regard, must not the issue of competence be settled independently of the frustrations met in caring for Amelda and of the possible benefits accruing to a more intelligent utilization of scarce medical resources?

(b) Legal Avenues to the Discontinuation of Treatment

(i) The health care professionals must try to reach agreement with each authority concerned. This would involve reaching agreement with the hospital authorities, all members of the health-care team, pathologists, and members of the family. If this approach were to be taken, it could require as many as twenty affidavits. Even if agreement could be reached, it would still be difficult to make a deal with the coroner in advance.

(ii) They can also take legal action by seeking court approval for the discontinuation of force-feeding.

(7) Moral Considerations

Amelda's case presents us with the following moral dilemma. If force-feeding is discontinued because it has been futile, health-care professionals may be contributing to Amelda's death; but if health-care professionals continue to force-feed her, in order to save her life, they will deny other more compliant patients essential treatment.

Neither alternative violates an ethical absolute. Contributing to the death of patients, in carefully defined circumstances, is not morally proscribed. Consider the case of John (Case 8:2) or a terminally-ill cancer patient who refuses chemotherapy, preferring to die. The patient's wishes are likely to be respected, even though they run counter to medical judgment. But Amelda is not terminal and has not expressed the wish to die. To be sure, her resistance to treatment is at odds with the verbal denials that she wishes to die. Indeed, this ambivalence may be traceable to her deficiency in insight and understanding, a deficiency that may be attributable to her illness.

The second alternative is also problematic. While it is true that the time, energy, and resources devoted to keeping Amelda alive might be better used to serve the needs of more compliant patients, can we follow a Kantian procedure and elevate to the status of a moral maxim the principle that medical resources be devoted only to the compliant? Clearly we are now in the domain of "value judgments" rather than strict "medical judgments." In considering the morality of not force-feeding Amelda, recall once again, Aristotle's description of moral life. Is cultivation and maintenance of the appropriate virtues consistent with a willingness to engage in selective starvation? Do we wish our health care professionals *to be* people who can do this sort of thing? Do *we* wish to be people who can sanction this kind of activity? On the other hand, is a willingness and ability to engage in such conduct any less consistent with maintaining virtue than discontinuing life-support? Perhaps the symbolic nature of nourishing a vulnerable person with food and water makes a difference. Perhaps not.

The view that we may sacrifice the lives of non-responsive patients to improve the quality of life of more responsive ones is underpinned by the notion that human lives are in some cases interchangeable – a notion that may be derived from the principle of utility, and which threatens many of the virtues upon which moral life is based. From the standpoint of cost/efficiency and a responsible distribution of scarce resources it is certainly preferable that patients with a more favourable prognosis be substituted for those with a less favourable outlook. But this presents serious ethical problems even in the context of a choice over whether to save one life rather than another when both cannot be saved. The problems become even more acute when one contemplates sacrificing the life of one patient in order to improve the quality of life of another. Again do we wish to *be* people who are willing to do this, even if the cost-benefit ratio is in its favour? Perhaps we should here heed the warnings of feminist theorists who stress the role of caring relationships and emotional commitment in moral life. Moral life requires caring more than it does calculation. Or is this a luxury we cannot afford when highly scarce resources are at issue?

Let us move now to the first premise of the dilemma. Here the term "futile" is ambiguous. While therapy has proved to be futile in terms of restoring Amelda's functioning and enabling her to fulfil roles associated with "normal" human beings, it has not proved to be futile in preserving her life.

The term "may" in "may contribute to her death" is chosen advisedly. When considering the discontinuation of force-feeding, one member of the health-care team suggested that this might have the force of throwing Amelda on her own resources and possibly setting her on the road to recovery. This suggestion meets with two difficulties. First, does Amelda have any resources? Second, whether such a dramatic recovery is a "remote possibility" or a "genuine probability" is open to question. If, on weighing the relevant factors, the balances are tipped in favour of "remote possibility," are we justified in playing a long shot when the stakes are so high – Amelda's life?

There is disagreement among Amelda's care-givers as to whether her resistance to treatment is an expression of self-will or of her illness. But where uncertainty exists, should we perhaps be on the safe side and attribute such reluctance to the patient's illness? Is that a defensible moral principle? Perhaps it is tempting to suppose that if Amelda has the will power to frustrate every effort of the medical profession to treat her, then she has the will power to get well. Unfortunately the matter is not that simple. Our wills may be the allies of our reasonable deliberation, or the slaves of our obsessional ideas. When the latter is true, is it realistic to suppose that the threat to stop force-feeding will help Amelda to snap out of her illness? If Amelda's resistance to treatment is pathological, then it is unrealistic to expect her to make a spectacular recovery. Is it not easy to succumb to a form of medical pessimism that announces, "If we can't make you well, we will let you die"? Is that a candidate for a guiding ethical principle?

The whole scenario is complicated by the fact that until now her condition has been treated as though it were pathological. Witness her certification at each admission, and remember that there has been no change in her status. Since this is so, is the drastic change in her treatment warranted? We are back at 6 (a) (iii) – "must not the issue of competence be settled independently of the frustrations met in caring for Amelda and the possible benefits accruing from a more intelligent use of scarce resources?"

The crux of the matter is that we find it easier to withhold treatment from those suffering from irreversible physical maladies than from those suffering from intractable mental illness. There comes a point in treating those suffering from physical ills when it no longer makes sense to pump any more blood into a vein or to keep the mechanical life-support systems going any longer (see, again, Case 8:2). But we experience great difficulty in calling a halt to treatment of the mentally-ill, even though we regard it as futile. Is this discrepancy capable of reasoned defence, or is it simply an expression of unanalyzed feeling? Perhaps the reasons go deeper in the present case because, in effect, we are comparing apples and oranges, life in one patient with quality of life in another.

Since quality of life enters into the reckoning we need to consider

(i) whether there are states of life worse than death; and (ii) whether Amelda is in such a state. For (i) we need acceptable criteria and for (ii) care needs to be exercised lest from our perspective of "normalcy" we project our own wishes on to Amelda.

Notes

1 Sidney Kennedy and Paul E. Garfinkel, "Anorexia Nervosa," *American Psychiatric Association Annual Review*, Vol. 4 (1986), 439.
2 Kennedy and Garfinkel, 442.
3 Claudia Wallace, "To Feed or not to Feed?" *Time* (March 31, 1986), 50.

Chapter 7: Esoteric Medicine

Case 7:1 A Baboon Heart for Baby Fae

On October 12, 1984, Baby Fae was born three weeks prematurely in a hospital in Barstow, California. It was clear from the beginning that something was seriously wrong. Doctors at the nearby Loma Linda University Medical Centre confirmed that Fae was suffering from hypoplastic left-heart syndrome, a fatal condition said to affect one in 12,000 newborns. In children with this affliction, the left side of the heart (including its main pumping chamber, the left ventricle, and the aorta) is seriously underdeveloped. Death normally occurs within two weeks of birth.

At Loma Linda, Fae's unwed mother, Teresa, was told that her daughter would probably die within a few days and that she could either leave her at the hospital or take her home. Teresa decided to take Fae home to die. But the hospital called within the next two days and offered Teresa the chance to save her daughter's life with a transplant from a baboon. Dr. Leonard Bailey, chief of paediatric heart surgery, had been experimenting for seven years with cross-species heart transplants involving sheep and goats, and had just recently received permission from the hospital research board to transplant a simian heart into a human infant. Although Fae would be the first infant to undergo such a procedure, she would not be the first human being to have done so. In 1964, a 68-year-old man's heart was replaced with that of a chimpanzee. He died within a few hours. In 1977, Christian Barnard, the South African transplant pioneer, made two attempts to implant the heart of a chimpanzee into a human patient. In each case the patient died very shortly after the operation. The odds against Fae's survival would be considerable. The immunological gap between humans and primates is very wide, though infants stand a better chance than mature adults. The need for anti-rejection drugs would be substantial and their use would create a strong risk of heart and kidney failure.

Teresa, together with Fae's father, from whom she was separated and who had in the meantime been contacted, accepted Dr. Bailey's offer. Each signed a reportedly elaborate, but unreleased, special consent form which had been prepared for the occasion. They then signed the form a required second time following a 20-hour period in which to reconsider their decision. According to the hospital, the parents were well informed of the risks and the alternatives.

On October 26 Fae's ailing heart was replaced with that of a healthy seven-month-old baboon. For two weeks following the operation, Fae was reported to be in serious but stable condition. On November 9, however, she showed the first signs of rejecting her new heart. On November 15 she died, apparently of complications stemming from the rejection episodes. Dr. Bailey had this to say on the occasion of her death, "Today we grieve the loss of this patient's life. Infants with heart disease yet to be born will some day have the opportunity to live, thanks to the courage of this infant and her parents. We are remarkably encouraged by what we have learned from Baby Fae."

Case Discussion

The case of Baby Fae sparked considerable public debate and controversy. In addition to general arguments concerning the optimal utilization of scarce resources (see Cases 7:3, 9:1, and 9:2), there were four other sources of concern in this particular case.

(1) Meddling with Nature

The transplantation of a simian heart into the breast of a human infant was thought by some to violate the natural order. Some people object to the bridging of any species, others only to the mixing of human with non-human. Such objections typically fall into two categories.

(a) It is feared that any violation of species barriers brings unacceptable risk of catastrophe. The extreme version of this fear suggests that we run the risk of creating a "monster" of the sort depicted in science fiction movies. Such concerns seem totally out of place here, however, where there is no intrusion into human reproduction but simply the replacing of an organ. (Even if reproduction were involved, a monster need not ensue – witness the case of horses and donkeys which have been successfully interbred to produce mules.) Monsters aside, there is fear of increasing the odds of rejection. The body's rejection of a foreign organ is a serious enough problem within species. Between species those risks may be considerably higher. To be sure, the risks to Fae were significant. But it is questionable whether they were any greater than those incurred by the first human heart transplant patients, who received their new organs without the bene-fit of cyclosporin-A, the relatively new, and effective, anti-rejection drug. It is also questionable whether Fae's chances were any worse than those of Barney Clark, the initial recipient of a permanent mechanical heart. So the mere fact that Fae's donor was of a different species seems not, in itself, to have meant that the risks were unac-ceptably high.

(b) There are some, however, who argue that bridging species bar-riers is wrong independently of potentially harmful consequences. It amounts to ghoulish tinkering, not morally responsible science. In their view, the human body has a uniqueness and sacredness which is violated by the invasion of foreign organs. But it is difficult to see why we should accept this point of view. Does it amount to anything more than simple "speciesism"? Would those who advance it be prepared to ban bovine insulin or the use of heart valves from pigs? Are these any less invasive than simian hearts?

(2) Animal Rights

Normally, transplant organs are offered willingly by the donor him-self or by someone empowered to do so on his behalf. In many juris-dictions, for example, automobile drivers may consent to the use of their organs by signing a form attached to their drivers' licences. And parents have the power to donate their children's organs. But in the case of Baby Fae, donor consent was not possible. A seven-month-old baboon, raised at Loma Linda, was simply selected to supply the desired organ. This raised the ire of various "animal rights" groups who protested the sacrifice of an animal for what they saw as scien-tifically dubious medical sensationalism. Michael Fox of the Humane Society's national office in Washington D.C. questioned whether it was proper to "put the burden for our suffering and that of our loved ones on the animal kingdom."[1] Leroy Walters, on the other hand, suggested that "It is regrettable that an animal has to be killed to allow a human a chance to live. But in a showdown, it is appropriate to come down on the side of saying 'let the human live'."[2]

Who is right here? May animals be used as "mere means" to the welfare of human beings? Should we be prepared to sacrifice an animal, however slight the chance that humans will benefit? Or can the Kantian injunction against using others as means to our own ends be extended to include animals, who are, after all, sentient creatures? May we sacrifice their lives only when the probability and degree of expected benefit for human beings are "sufficiently great"? But how do we determine a sufficient level of expected benefit? And was it surpassed in the case of Baby Fae? Could the transplant properly be described as the immoral sacrifice of a sentient creature for reasons of "medical sensationalism"?

(3) The Alternatives

Some physicians challenged the propriety of using an animal heart when a human organ would have been much more suitable. It was not clear that alternative procedures had been seriously considered. When it became known on the day of Fae's operation that the heart of a human infant was available for transplant, Loma Linda Hospital officials reportedly "admitted that they simply had not considered the possibility of a human donor."[3] "They said that the hospital did not have a human heart transplant program, and that Bailey had been wholly concerned with demonstrating the feasibility of using baboons as donors."[4]

In fairness to Bailey and his colleagues, it must be noted that on the day of her transplant, Fae was on the brink of death. Hence there was no time to check for donor compatibility and to transport the newly available human organ. By then the options were to implant the baboon heart or let Fae die. In addition, we must consider the claim by Loma Linda surgeon David Hinshaw that, "his colleagues believed that the hope of finding a compatible human heart in time to save the dying Fae was 'almost nonexistent'."[5] Indeed, the extreme scarcity of infant donors is what principally motivated Dr. Bailey to seek to establish his new procedure.

Nevertheless, the hospital's comments strongly suggest that Bailey and his colleagues had never really considered seriously the possibility of finding a suitable human heart at any stage following Fae's birth.

To be sure, the odds of finding one were not great, and the Loma Linda surgeons would themselves have been unable, for lack of official authorization, to perform the required surgery. But there was a chance that a suitable heart could be found, and there were other institutions authorized to transplant human hearts. Was it not Loma Linda's duty to pursue these options vigorously before they resorted to a much riskier, highly experimental procedure? Or was their obligation only to provide the best care they *themselves* could provide?

Of equal importance was the presence of another option which again seems not to have been seriously considered. Many physicians commented on the availability of a form of corrective surgery for hypoplastic heart which had been developed by Dr. William Norwood of the Children's Hospital of Philadelphia. Norwood's procedure was being practised at a small number of hospitals in the United States and involved rerouting blood through the heart so that the right ventricle could assume the pumping function normally performed by the left ventricle. According to Norwood, 40 of the 100 infants he had treated with this procedure had survived. The oldest was, at that time, four.

The case of Baby Fae serves as a vivid illustration of the conflict between physician as therapist and physician as investigator. Where precisely did Dr. Bailey's loyalties and interests lie? Was he more concerned with establishing the viability of his new procedure than with Baby Fae? Was he willing to trade off the welfare of his patient and her family for the sake of scientific knowledge and the welfare of future patients? Was he morally entitled to do so? Is a physician entitled to pursue a riskier "therapy" for the sake of a possible greater good? Even if the "physician" may take this line, may he do so without properly informing the patient or her surrogates of the alternative options? Did Fae and her parents have a right to know which hat Bailey was wearing – that of physician or that of researcher?

(4) Informed Consent

Loma Linda's admission that they had never considered a human heart transplant raised worries about the extent to which Fae's parents had been apprised of the available options. These worries were further fuelled by public statements by Dr. Bailey in which he "understated the success rate" of the Norwocd procedure, and by the hospital's refusal to make public the consent form signed by Fae's parents.[6]

So we might question whether consent was truly informed.

Of further concern was whether consent was fully voluntary. Were Fae's parents "enticed" by Loma Linda's offer to pay all the expenses involved in the transplant? They were poor in a country without universal medical insurance, and had recently separated. Without the means of pursuing more promising options at other institutions (assuming they were aware of them), the temptation to accept Loma Linda's offer must have been almost overwhelming. Their only other viable option was to accept the death of their newborn child. Was it morally responsible for Bailey and his colleagues to have extended the offer they did? What was offered appears not to have been the best available therapy but a less promising experimental procedure which they, as scientific investigators, had a stake in pursuing. Does this fact render their offer morally questionable? Did they in effect exploit the natural inclination of people in such situations to grasp at any straw, however slender? Or were they only offering a charitable hand to a trio of individuals in desperate need of their help? Bailey found it hard to understand why people would question a potentially life-saving procedure. "If you had the opportunity to see this baby and her mother together, and see this baby in the best shape she's ever been, you would see the propriety of what we are doing," he said shortly before Fae died.[7] But compare the following comment by Professor Albert Johnson, also made shortly before Fae's death, "If this infant matches the best transplant record in the world – Stanford's, with 50 per cent five-year survival – what will her five years be like? Her loving parents, who would have lost a baby, will lose a child."[8]

Notes

1 *Newsweek*, November 12, 118.

2 *Newsweek*.

3 *Time*, November 12, 1984.

4 *Facts on File*, 1984, 866.

5 *Time*, November 12, 1984.

6 *Time*, November 26, 1984,86.

7 *Time*, November 12, 1984, 64.

8 *Hamilton Spectator*, November 5, 1984.

Case 7:2 Did Family Instability Justify Non-Treatment of Baby Jesse?

Jesse was born at Huntington Memorial Hospital in Pasadena, California on May 25, 1986. He, like Baby Fae, was diagnosed as having hypoplastic left-heart syndrome. Jesse was given three hours to two weeks to live. Following the discovery of his condition, the hospital referred Jesse's parents to Loma Linda University Medical Centre and placed him on medication in preparation for an eventual human heart transplant.

At Loma Linda, Jesse's parents were interviewed by the hospital's heart transplant screening committee. The committee discovered that the parents were young and unwed. According to newspaper reports the father was a 26-year-old employed by an air conditioning and heating company "who had a record of arrests for drunk driving and had been through a 'substance abuse' treatment program."[1] The mother was a 17-year-old. The parents reportedly informed the committee that "before the child's birth, they considered putting him up for adoption because they doubted they were ready to be parents."[2] But according to Right-to-Life spokeswoman Susan McMillan, who together with Father Michael Carcerano brought Jesse's plight to international attention, the young couple's intention was "impulsive" and was quickly abandoned once Jesse was born. Carcerano claimed that the couple were now "committed to keeping and caring for Jesse."[3]

Upon completion of the interview, Jesse was turned down for a transplant. Loma Linda officials declined, for reasons of confidentiality, to give details of the criteria used by the screening committee. Following the rejection, family members approached Carcerano and the anti-abortion group, who eventually discovered that Loma Linda was reluctant to commit its resources to a child whose family life did not seem stable enough to provide necessary postoperative care. "Young transplant patients require constant monitoring for rejection, lifelong medication, and special precautions to avoid infection."[4] The committee's reluctance was publicly endorsed by a spokesman for the adult heart transplantation program at Stanford University who said: "If the patient does not have a stable situation at home, all that has been accomplished is to subject him to a highly invasive operation with a lessened chance that he will recover."[5]

McMillan disagreed. At a press conference she said, "We had an outrageous violation of civil rights here."[6] The ensuing public outcry led Loma Linda to agree to a deal. Jesse would be placed on the Regional Procurement Agency List, if legal custody were surrendered to his grandparents. The agreement called for custody to remain with the grandparents till the completion of treatment. On June 5 the transfer was made and Jesse was put on the waiting list. In an official statement, the hospital said that "responsibility for continuing care ... has been transferred from his parents to his paternal grandparents." With the assurance of "reliable care for the baby," they added, "the committee has recommended that Baby Jesse be considered eligible for cardiac transplantation."[7] McMillan's husband, Bill, an attorney who arranged the transfer of custody, expressed the following doubt, "I don't know whether custody will ever be relinquished [to the young parents]."[8]

On June 17, Jesse's parents appeared on Phil Donohue's TV talk show to make a public plea for a human heart. During the course of that program, a call was placed to Butterworth Hospital in Grand Rapids, Michigan. A spokeswoman for the hospital was persuaded to reveal that they had located a suitable donor. Frank Clemenshaw, 22, and Deborah Walters, 33, had been moved by the public pleas of Jesse's parents to donate the heart of their brain-dead child. Eventually, Jesse was successfully implanted with the donor heart.

Should the social status of patients determine the allocation of scarce medical resources? And is it right to "go public" with one's case as Jesse's parents did?

Case Discussion

(1) The Initial Decision

The case of Baby Fae concerned the moral and/or clinical propriety of a new, highly experimental procedure. There were reasons to think that the risks incurred in that procedure were too high and that other, more promising, options deserved greater consideration. With Jesse, on the other hand, the key issue was not the adequacy of a new type of treatment but the proper allocation of a generally accepted form of therapy. Precisely how should we determine the beneficiaries of our scarce, life-saving resources?

In its decision-making, the Loma Linda screening committee

invoked a curious blend of two competing allocation criteria: (a) social status and (b) medical benefit. Normally (b) involves judgments concerning the physiological status of the patient. Does his blood type match sufficiently that of the donor? Will his cancer kill him anyway, even if we give him a new heart? And so on. But physiological considerations apparently played no role in the thinking of the committee. Jesse's ability to benefit medically hinged, not on his bodily status, but on the social status of his parents. They were a young, unwed couple, one of whom had a record of drug abuse and arrests for drunk driving. They were financially unstable and had earlier expressed anxiety about raising a (normal) child. In the view of the committee, these "social" factors were sufficient indication that Jesse would not receive essential postoperative care. And without such care, he could in no way benefit medically from a heart transplant.

The burning question, then, is whether social criteria should in this way determine or influence allocation decisions. Should doctors stick to what they know best – physiological indications? Or may they look at the wider social picture? Loma Linda's reasons for inclining toward the latter option were fairly clear and straightforward. They were dealing with a very scarce, potentially life-saving resource whose effectiveness greatly depends on social factors. Were they to ignore such factors, they would be guilty of squandering a precious resource. Jesse's surgeon, Dr. Leonard Bailey, put the point this way, "You can't serve up hearts like cherries jubilee...."[9]

Nevertheless, there are at least four objections to assigning social elements this important role in micro-allocation decisions. First, there is the immense difficulty in predicting whether essential post-operative care will be provided or accepted willingly by patients in general. Consider the potential adult heart-transplant patient who has a poor record of following doctor's orders, or who generally acts in defiance of authority. Can we assume that his "bad" habits will continue? Or can we sometimes reasonably expect a new leaf to be turned, especially when the only other option is certain death? Should such predictive difficulties make us wary of ever departing from purely physiological criteria?

Secondly, there is the spectre of abuse. Social criteria may often be interpreted and applied in a variety of ways. They are "highly subjective," "matters of opinion." It may thus be possible for a committee, unwittingly or not, to "rationalize" its decision to withhold treatment, to deny access not because the patient is *incapable* of benefitting but because he is judged *unworthy* of doing so. When widened to include social elements, "ability to benefit medically" may too easily be translated into "perceived social worth."

Of related concern is the issue of fairness. If social criteria are highly pliable, then we face the possibility that equals will be treated unequally, or unequals equally. This, as Aristotle pointed out long ago, is the essence of injustice. Our decisions may turn out to be arbitrary, and hence unjust to those denied.

Abuses aside, there is a fourth reason for caution. Decisions based on social criteria may be an affront to the dignity of persons. Is it morally permissible to withhold life-saving treatment because a person's social situation renders him a "bad investment"? Especially if his investment potential is a function not of his own weaknesses, mistakes, and misfortunes, but of those of his parents?

Compare here the decision of Canada and of many European countries to remove basic education and health care from the marketplace and to opt instead for universal access at no direct cost to the individual. In these countries ability to pay has been deemed an unacceptable basis upon which to allocate vital resources. Need alone determines allocation. And we need not look far for the reason. Ability to pay is largely a function of fortuitous factors (e.g. accident of birth) over which we have little control; it is *prima facie* unfair to base the satisfaction of vital needs on such factors. But did Loma Linda not do just that when it turned Jesse down? *His* ability to benefit medically was no less a function of fortuitous factors than the ability of his parents to pay. Was this an affront to his dignity as a human, a dignity which cannot be reduced to a matter of social status? Do we not here reach a point where human dignity cannot be traded off for utility?

(2) The Compromise

In the end, Jesse was placed on the waiting list, but only after custody was surrendered to the paternal grandparents. Was this an acceptable compromise – or a coercive measure? One's answer will depend, presumably, on whether one accepts Loma Linda's grounds for rejecting Jesse. If social criteria are judged unacceptable, then the compromise must be condemned; it is based on those very same criteria. If, on the other hand, we accept social criteria, then we will view the compromise in an entirely different light. It not only qualified Jesse for the transplant and improved his chances considerably, but also did so without removing him entirely from the care of his (extended) family. Compared with the alternatives – certain death or his being made a ward of the state – this option may have had considerable merit.

(3) The Media

The media played a major role in Jesse's story. It was they who brought the story to international attention and arguably forced Loma Linda's hand. They were also instrumental in securing the donor heart. The Michigan couple who donated their child's heart "admitted they had been moved to do so by televised reports on Jesse and his parents. 'Our baby could not live,' said [the mother], whose son was brain-dead at birth. 'We'd seen their plea on TV, and we figured that if our baby could help them, then it would not be a total loss.'"[10]

All this raises questions concerning the media's power to determine who receives donor organs. To be sure, without their help Jesse might have died. But what do we say to those in equal need whose stories failed to make the evening news? A case in point: Baby Calvin had been waiting longer than Jesse for a heart. His parents had "elected to work quietly through organ-procurement networks rather than seek publicity for their child.... At present, they charged, 'it almost seems like publicity is the only method that's working.'"[11] Fortunately, another donor was found and Calvin had his transplant. But the question still remains: should our allocation criteria be found in media publicity and sensationalism? Or should the kind of "queue-jumping" this allows be prohibited?

Notes

1   *Time*, June 23, 1986.
2   *The Los Angeles Times*, June 4, 1986.
3   *LA Times*, June 4, 1986
4   *Time*, June 23, 1986.
5   *LA Times*, June 4, 1986.
6   *Time*, June 23, 1986.
7   *LA Times*, June 6, 1986.
8   *LA Times*, June 6, 1986
9   *Time*, June 23, 1986.
10 *Time*, June 23, 1986.
11 *Time*, June 23, 1986.

Case 7:3 A Jarvik-7 Heart: Experiment or Therapy?

On November 25, 1984, William Schroeder became the world's second recipient of a permanent artificial heart. The first, in 1982, was Dr. Barney Clark, who survived for 112 days. Schroeder, a 52-year-old native of Jasper, Illinois, had been suffering from terminal arteriosclerosis. Until two years previously, he had lived a normal, active life, his only health problem being a case of diabetes which had been successfully controlled through diet. In January of 1983, however, Schroeder suffered a massive heart attack which seriously damaged his heart. By the fall of 1984 he was largely bedridden and unable to walk more than a few feet without chest pain and shortness of breath.

Under normal circumstances, Schroeder would have been a candidate for a human heart transplant, but he was excluded because of his age and his diabetes. According to Dr. J.P. Salb, Schroeder's family physician, were Schroeder to receive a transplant, "the antirejection drugs would just throw his diabetes out of control."[1] His only hope was an artificial heart, which would avoid rejection problems. On the suggestion of his physician and cardiologist, and with the support of his family, Schroeder was admitted to Humana Hospital. Humana agreed to pay for the $15,500 heart and its drive system, to supply free accommodation within the hospital for the entire Schroeder family, and to provide the patient with a specially designed house should he become well enough to leave the hospital. Bearing in mind that Barney Clark's hospital bill alone had been $200,000, Humana's financial commitment was considerable.

Schroeder and his family were reportedly informed of the risks of the procedure, and provided with a 17-page consent form indicating, among other things, all the medical difficulties encountered by Barney Clark. These included brain seizures and serious depression. "The last was included because Clark had complained to psychiatrists that he wanted to die, that his 'mind was shot...'"[2]

The implant operation was performed by Clark's surgeon, Dr. William DeVries, the only person authorized by the American Food and Drug Administration to undertake the procedure. In the words of Schroeder's surgeons, the procedure had gone "almost routinely."[3]

Four days after the Jarvik-7 heart had been implanted, Schroeder got out of bed, walked several steps, and enjoyed a can of Coors beer. In December, however, things began to take a turn for the worse. Schroeder suffered a stroke that left him with severely impaired speech and memory problems. On February 18, 1985, Dr. Allan Lansing, chief medical spokesman for the artificial heart program, reported that Schroeder "was 'weak, tired, and discouraged,' suffering from an unexplained fever, and might never leave the hospital."[4] Clark had also complained "that he found it enormously disappointing to wake up and find that he was still alive with the artificial heart pounding away in his chest."[5] By February 20 he was said to be improving and on March 12 he tied Barney Clark's survival record.

On April 6, Schroeder became the first artificial heart patient to leave the hospital when he was moved to the specially equipped house supplied by Humana. He was readmitted on May 6 after suffering a brain haemorrhage. In the May issue of *Life Magazine*, Schroeder's wife, Margaret, claimed that she was "no longer so hopeful about her husband's prospects. 'I see it as more of a research experiment,' she said. 'The longer he lives, the more information [doctors] will get. Only for us it's so hard sometimes.'"[6]

On November 11, 1985, Schroeder suffered a third stroke and was reported to be in serious condition. The haemorrhage had occurred in an area of his brain unaffected by the earlier strokes. Hospital officials claimed that he "was able to speak a few single-syllable words and to move his arms and legs."[7] William Schroeder died on August 6, 1986.

Case Discussion

In discussing Fae and Jesse we centred on micro-allocation issues concerning the conditions under which individual patients have access to scarce medical resources. The present case raises many of these same issues. In addition, however, it raises serious questions of macro-allocation; these will serve as our focus.

Macro decision-making concerns the initiation and maintenance of medical programs and services. Such decisions do not directly concern individuals, but large, impersonal, statistical groups. This level of decision-making presents two closely related questions:

(1) What resources shall we devote to health care as opposed to other social goods (e.g. education, work-programs, community recreation, improving the environment, a minimally decent postal system, and defence)?

(2) Within the area of health care and once we have answered question (1) what resources shall we allocate to which programs?

Heart transplants prompt serious thought about both these questions. It has been estimated in the United States that 50,000 persons per year could benefit from artificial or transplanted hearts.[8] In Canada, given comparable backgrounds and life-styles, the corresponding number would likely be 5,000. At an estimated average cost per operation of roughly $150,000 (in 1984 U.S. dollars) the price of these services, were they to become generally available, would amount to a staggering sum. In light of these prohibitive costs, the question arises as to whether our dollars would be better spent elsewhere.

(1) Health-Care Versus Other Social Goods

We should begin by noting the limited role medical care has generally played in improving our health.[9] In particular, our exotic medical technologies have offered only marginal returns in reducing illness and premature death. Other factors seem to have been at least as effective: improvements in living conditions, better air, improved sanitation, more conscientious life-styles, and so on. Thus the pursuit of these other social goods might well prove to be more cost-efficient than more sophisticated medical techniques.

This observation notwithstanding, it cannot be denied that medical care does play a significant role in improving our lives. So we must still decide how much of our resources it warrants. In making this decision we confront a fundamental conflict between the value of health care and other social goods. Should hospitals always take precedence over museums, public parks, opera houses, and hockey rinks?

An affirmative answer to this latter question is often based on a version of the following argument: "*Basic needs* are essential to human flourishing regardless of what we, as individuals, choose to do with our lives. Without their satisfaction, nothing else of value in life is possible. Health, along with such things as basic shelter and food, qualifies as a basic need. As the old saying goes, without one's health one has nothing. Mere *wants*, on the other hand, are for things inessential to human flourishing, but which add *quality* to our lives. There are many things we desperately want and without which our lives would be impoverished; but we can do without them. The result is that mere wants are far less urgent than basic needs, and in cases of conflict must always bow to them. It follows that we must always choose improved medical care over museums and hockey rinks."

This argument has considerable appeal, but there are at least two reasons to question its soundness. First, we might ask whether all that goes on in the name of improved medical care serves the basic human need to be free of incapacitating disease and premature death. Perhaps a good deal of medical activity serves to promote a (non-basic) wish to enrich the quality of our lives. Consider, for example, cosmetic surgery, plastic surgery to restore a burn victim's facial features, or costly efforts to circumvent infertility. If these (and many other) forms of medical activity serve only to enrich our lives, then it seems as though medical care sometimes competes on an equal footing with other non-essential social goods.

Secondly, we might question the premise that basic needs have absolute priority over mere wants. A society that allows people to die from preventable disease is no doubt one we should wish to avoid. We would not want to be such people. But a community without theatres, symphony halls, festivals, public parks, or hockey rinks would impoverish us in other ways. Is it obvious that these "non-essential" social goods must never be pursued if we have yet to achieve a perfectly healthy society? Many of the governments of post-Second-World-War Europe did not think so. They were prepared to allocate a portion of their resources to help restore cultural institutions and churches which had been devastated by the war, resources which could have been used in the ongoing restoration of homes and hospitals. Were these policies immoral?

(2) Priorities in Health-Care

We now come to the macro-allocation question most directly related to William Schroeder. Should our health care dollars be spent on developing costly mechanical hearts which benefit a relatively small number of people? Many will answer negatively, arguing that our money is more efficiently and fairly spent in other less glamorous ways. We can expect a far greater return on our investment and benefit a far greater number of people if we concentrate on such things as early detection of disease, more frequent examinations, health education, modification of life-style, better hospitals, more community clinics, and so on. According to Rita Spence, president of Emerson

Hospital in Concord, Massachusetts, the bill for William Schroeder's operation "represents 790 days of hospital care at her hospital, or full treatment for 113 patients for an average stay of a week. 'That's what is in the balance.'"[10]

But we must also factor into the equation possible future spin-offs of costly experimental procedures. Many currently standard therapies which benefit a great number of people were once condemned as extravagant, the cardiac pacemaker and the artificial kidney, to name two. Commenting on the artificial heart, Dr. Michael Hess of the Medical College of Virginia said, "This is a case of spending money on research that will be useful in the future. Only God knows when the future is in this profession, but you have to start somewhere."[11]

So from a purely consequentialist or utilitarian perspective, the approach to be taken in answering question (2) is clear. We must somehow weigh short term losses against possible long term gains. What is not so clear is whether we have the means with which to make the comparison, especially if "only God knows the future." But there may be other non-consequentialist factors which complicate the picture even further, factors such as the symbolic value of the policies we adopt and what those policies say about us as moral agents. According to James Childress, "rescue attempts show that individuals are 'priceless' and that society is 'too good' to let them die without great efforts to save them... Allocation policies may be thought of as ways for society to define and express its sense of itself, its values, and its integrity."[12] On this view, with which feminists and Aristotelians will have great sympathy, we should worry about a society capable of allowing a William Schroeder to die without pursuing all possible efforts to save him.

Nevertheless, some will question whether this view is rationally and morally defensible. Should we really, for reasons such as the symbolic value of our policies, favour the few in present peril over the future many who could benefit more from a wiser allocation of resources? One of the primary elements in practical prudence, what Aristotle called *phronesis*, is the ability and willingness to think not solely in terms of the dramatic and the here and now, but also in terms of long range consequences and possibilities. Is the same not true of morality? Is our present tendency to invest in rescue interventions like artificial hearts and dialysis machines, as opposed to less dramatic but more efficient health care programs, a function not of sound moral thinking, but of an irrational inclination to discount what is not presently before our eyes? Or is this an area where the limits of rationality are encountered and compassion must determine our choices? Once again, do we want to be a society for whom such displays of "rationality" are not fully determinative of our choices?

Notes

1   *Time*, December 10, 1984.
2   *Time.*
3   *Facts on File*, November 30, 1984.
4   *Facts on File*, March 1, 1985.
5   *Time*, December 10, 1984.
6   *Facts on File,* March 1, 1985, 350.
7   *Facts on File*, December. 6, 1985.
8   "One Miracle, Many Doubts,'" *Time*, December 10, 1984.
9   J.F. Mustard, "Population Health and Health Care," in J.E. Thomas (ed.), *Medical Ethics and Human Life* (Toronto: Samuel Stevens & Co., 1983).
10   "One Miracle," note 1.
11   "One Miracle."
12   James Childress, "Priorities in the Allocation of Health Care Resources," *Soundings* 62 (Fall, 1979).

Chapter 8: Death, Dying, and Euthanasia

Case 8:1 "Don't Let My Mother Die"

Mrs. Jones was an 81-year-old woman who lived in Edmonton with her son. She had no other relatives in Canada except for a small number of grandchildren who lived in Calgary. Though Mrs. Jones had spent a fair bit of time in Canada, she was a native Jamaican and identified very closely with her homeland and its traditions. For over a year Mrs. Jones had suffered great deterioration in her health. She had, in the preceding few months, undergone several cardio-respiratory arrests. The cause of these attacks was diagnosed as paralysis of her breathing muscles. Mrs. Jones had several months before been placed on a respirator, and several attempts to wean her from the machine had met with unmitigated failure. There was no question that if Mrs. Jones were taken off the respirator, she would die very quickly from oxygen starvation. Her attending physicians all concurred that Mrs. Jones would in all likelihood suffer further cardiac arrests, despite any efforts to control them, and that there was no possibility of restoring her breathing muscles.

Mrs. Jones had been in the ICU (the Intensive Care Unit) for several weeks. She was at this stage only semi-conscious, almost totally unaware of her surroundings and incapable of rational discussion. In the opinion of her attending physicians, Mrs. Jones was incapable now of informed consent. There was, therefore, no possibility of consulting Mrs. Jones to determine whether, in her present condition, she wished to be resuscitated in the event of further cardiac arrest. However, Mrs. Jones's son made it clear that both he and his mother were deeply religious and were firmly committed to the belief that, should his mother die in a foreign land – i.e., not in Jamaica – her soul would be condemned to wander the universe aimlessly for an eternity. He also made it clear that, before she lapsed into semi-consciousness, his mother had placed upon him a "conditional curse" which was to take effect if he failed to secure her return to Jamaica before she died. It should be stressed that the son took this curse very seriously. He therefore insisted quite adamantly that his mother's death be postponed as long as possible so that he could arrange for her return to Jamaica. However, the son was both penniless and unemployed with no immediate prospects of finding a job. As a result he lacked completely the means to fulfil his mother's wishes. The hospital pursued the possibility of provincial funding for transport to Jamaica but encountered a bureaucratic brick wall. Alberta Health Care's policy is to foot transportation costs only when essential medical treatment is unavailable in Alberta but can be found elsewhere. A further complication was the son's threat to kill the doctors should they not pursue every available avenue to postpone his mother's death.

Given these unusual and tragic circumstances, the attending physicians were perplexed. Their question was whether a DNR (Do-Not-Resuscitate) order should be issued, despite the son's vigorous protests.

Case 8:2 "Please Let Me Die"

This case is in many respects different from the preceding one. John was not an elderly patient near death, but rather a young man of 26 afflicted with a neurological disease commonly known as "the elephant man's disease." The disease manifests itself in non-malignant tumours which attach themselves to the body's nerves, often causing severe disfigurement (as in the case of the nineteenth-century Englishman John Merrick, after whom the disease is named) and radical impairment of bodily functions. John's illness was diagnosed at the age of seven and he had therefore suffered with the disease for 20 years. He had, over the course of his lifetime, undergone well over a hundred operations to remove tumours. The end results of these surgical interventions were: (1) total deafness and partial blindness; (2) total paralysis except for slight movement in the right shoulder; (3) total impairment of the breathing muscles, with the consequence that John, like Mrs. Jones, was a captive of the respirator; (4) a feeling of having been mutilated by the countless surgical procedures; and (5) a demand by John that no more surgery be undertaken. The attending surgeon testified that, in his view, John had tumours growing on every nerve in his body, and that there was no chance of remission. All the medical personnel and social workers who had been involved with the case were of the opinion that, despite his almost total physical debilitation and severe depression, John was fully alert, conscious, and in control of his mental faculties. He was able clearly to make rational decisions and choices. One of his choices was that no more be done to prolong his life and that he be disconnected from the respirator. In simple terms, he wanted to die.

John's family were stunned by his request and were at first strongly opposed. In time, however, and after numerous sessions with counsellors, they reluctantly agreed that John's request should be honoured and the respirator turned off. According to the physicians involved in John's case, were the respirator turned off John would in all likelihood die within a few hours from oxygen starvation, though as the case of Karen Ann Quinlan has shown, there are no certainties in such matters. They testified further that, were life support continued, John would probably live for many years. Nonetheless, they were prepared: (1) to disconnect life support; (2) to administer medication which would narcotize John, thus making the dying process less painful and distressful; but (3) they were not prepared to administer an amount of medication which could in any way accelerate John's death. In short, they were prepared to allow, but not hasten, death.

Case Discussions

(1) Sanctity of Life vs. Quality of Life

Perhaps the first question should be whether non-resuscitation or the withdrawal of life-support is even an option. Should doctors be in the business of allowing or causing the death of patients? Those who espouse the extreme version of the "sanctity of human life" argument will answer this question negatively, arguing that human life in all of its forms, at all of its stages, and regardless of its "quality," has a special, inestimable worth or value which places upon us all the absolute duty to preserve and protect it whenever we can. This duty would clearly be violated if no attempt were made to resuscitate Mrs. Jones, or if John were disconnected from his respirator. Others, such as Warren and Fletcher, locate the special value of human lives in qualities or properties normally associated with "persons," like rationality, self-awareness, and autonomy.[1] Only when a human life has these distinctive qualities does it have that special value which is the foundation of our duty to preserve and protect it whenever possible.

Vigorously pursued, the sanctity of life approach provides easy solutions to our practical difficulties. We must not disconnect John from his respirator and we must make every effort to resuscitate Mrs. Jones. Easy solutions, however, are purchased at a price. We need to ask whether the sanctity principle is relevant in all cases. Take John, for instance. Here was a man who was woefully lacking in most of the capacities which enrich the lives of human beings. Do we really want to say that respect for the sanctity of John's life requires that we take all conceivable steps to preserve his existence – even against his expressed wishes? An affirmative answer is not a foregone conclusion. Paradoxically, respect for John's life may be better expressed in respecting his wish to die. There is little, if anything, left in John's life which *he* values. The "quality of his life," as seen through his own eyes, is all but gone. Yet perhaps there is something of value left in John's life so long as we, or John's family, do not attempt to undermine it for paternalistic or self-interested reasons. We refer, of course, to John's autonomy, his normative power to determine the course of his own medical treatment. Perhaps we respect the special worth, even the "sanctity," of John's life by allowing him what little autonomy he has left, by allowing him death by *his* choice, not the choice of *others*, we who might be strongly tempted to exert our control over his life.

If, on the other hand, we reject the sanctity principle, we are left with a host of other problems. Were we to suppose, for example, that our special duty to preserve and protect human life extends only to the lives of human *persons*, not human *beings*, then we would in some way have to determine whether Mrs. Jones falls within that moral category. Note that she lacks all the qualities listed by Warren and Fletcher. Does this mean that Mrs. Jones the person, not the human biological organism with which that person might have once been associated, no longer exists? Or does "enough" of her personality exist to say that she is a person whose life we must attempt to preserve? Should we even be asking such questions? Does this case serve to illustrate the dangers of giving up the sanctity of life principle?

(2) Interests, Wishes, and Consent

Consider now the role of the patient's wishes. Consent was clearly lacking in Mrs. Jones's case. The son was vehemently opposed to the non-resuscitation order and it is reasonable to suppose that Mrs. Jones, had she been competent, would have objected as well. We could not, with justification, ascribe hypothetical, indirect or constructive consent to her. So many of the usual problems surrounding consent did not arise. The patient's wishes were clear and these in no way conflicted with those of her son. In addition, there was no question of imposing unwanted medical treatment on grounds of the patient's best interests – the classic interests vs. wishes dilemma. Rather the issue reduces to whether treatment could be *withdrawn* despite the wishes of both patient and family.

Underlying this question is a more fundamental one whose answer has very broad implications: Do we have a moral right – a positive right – to be provided, upon demand, with whatever treatment the medical establishment is capable of providing? This would be a right which holds so long as we, in our own person or through the actions of our agent, do not exercise our power to waive it. Consider in this context such things as heart transplants or kidney dialysis, discussed in Chapters 7 and 9. Do we have a moral right to these things whenever they are available? Or is our right limited, even non-existent? Recall Mrs. Jones. She was virtually comatose, and dying with no hope of recovery. Barring a miracle, there was no chance of her wish to die in Jamaica being fulfilled. The only question concerned the timing of her death. Is it obvious that efforts should have been made to prolong the dying process?

One's initial inclination may be to say yes, if only for the sake of the son. Regardless of the general tenability of his unorthodox religious beliefs, they did have a profound impact on his life, and his distress would be considerable were the DNR order issued. Compare our reactions to the Jehovah's Witness who declines a blood transfusion on grounds which are no less unorthodox. If we are willing to respect his idiosyncratic wishes regardless of their apparent irrationality, then should we not do the same for Mrs. Jones and her son?

Perhaps not. It may be one thing to respect idiosyncratic *refusals* of potentially life-saving treatment, and quite another to respect *demands* for such treatment based on unreasonable or eccentric beliefs. In the former case we not only honour the patient's right to refuse treatment, we save valuable resources for patients who desperately want and need them. In the latter case, however, we diminish our resources. Intensive medical care of the sort required to sustain Mrs. Jones is a very scarce and expensive resource. Is it clear that Mrs.

Jones – or her son – is entitled to a share of that resource, given that it can in no way serve a therapeutic or curative function, but only postpone impending death? If we continue to answer affirmatively, then what do we say to the patient who can genuinely benefit from the ICU and who may be denied access because a respirator is being used to sustain Mrs. Jones's biological existence? Would we be guilty of an injustice towards him? Or is this an area where the limits of rationality are again met and compassion must reign instead? What would refusal to sustain Mrs. Jones say about us as moral agents? Do we wish to be the kind of people who are willing and able to withdraw support from a dying human being who has requested it? Do we wish our health care professionals to be of this nature?

With John we have a quite different issue of consent. Here the question is whether, in the presence of an informed, express wish on the part of the patient that life-sustaining treatment be discontinued, doctors must comply. Does the patient have the power of veto over a physician's judgment that such treatment is medically indicated? And what about the patient's family? Recall that John's family were initially opposed to the withdrawal of support. It was only after extensive counselling that they were brought to accept his decision. What should the role of the counsellor be here? Should she serve as patient advocate, one who defends the patient's expressed wishes, whatever these might be? Or must she instead, or in addition, serve the patient's best interests and perhaps those of his family? May she actually attempt to persuade family members that their loved one's wishes should be respected, even when that wish is for death?

(3) The Dying and the Non-Dying

With Mrs. Jones we have an elderly person who is pretty clearly dying, with no hope of recovery. The question here is whether that process should be prolonged and death delayed, even though the delay will not serve the purpose for which it was requested. John, however, is quite clearly not dying. Does this make a moral difference? Is it permissible to shorten the life of a dying patient but impermissible to do the same when the patient is not yet dying?[2] There is some plausibility in viewing the matter in the following way. Whether a patient is dying or not, it remains true that he is still alive. And so we must still decide whether his life, regardless of its likely duration, must be preserved. What difference does it make whether the life is soon to be ended, or whether the forces of death are actively at work against it? If that life has whatever special value we ascribe to the lives of human persons, and which thereby imposes upon us special duties to preserve and protect it, then it has that value. Our duties towards it are the same as our duties towards the lives of people who are not yet in the throes of death. Whether the patient is soon to die seems totally irrelevant. Or is there something missing here?

(4) Active and Passive Measures

This brings us to an issue which is of great concern to medical practitioners. Is there a morally relevant difference between (a) not taking steps to resuscitate a patient, with the knowledge that one's intervention could prevent her death; and (b) actually taking steps, like turning off a respirator or administering life-shortening medication, with knowledge that one's steps will result in the death, or the accelerated death, of a patient? According to many people, and to the law, there is a very great difference between (a) and (b). In the view of others,[3] however, there is no such difference. Permitting some other force to do its work when one easily could, and normally would intervene, is no different, morally speaking, from serving as the active force oneself. In each case, the end of death has been chosen, regardless of the means of its achievement. Are the means a matter of indifference?

Lawrence Becker thinks not. Much as Aristotle might have done, Becker argues that good health care professionals must develop dispositions and personality traits which are totally at variance with killing, but not necessarily with giving up to the forces of death. Killing is inconsistent with the dispositions of good health care professionals because it is "complicitous with the processes they are committed to combating" – death and disease.[4] Doctors who allow patients to die merely surrender to the enemy. Those who kill patients actually serve him.

Even if there is a difference between killing and letting die, whether it warrants drawing a sharp moral and legal distinction between turning off John's respirator and not resuscitating Mrs. Jones is debatable. Consider in this regard Anthony Shaw's description[5] of what sometimes happens when doctors and parents decide not to operate on defective newborns and to "let them die" instead. According to James Rachels, a doctrine that says that a baby may be allowed in this way to dehydrate and wither, but may not be given an injection that would end its life without suffering, "seems so patently cruel as to require no further refutation."[6] If this is true, then we might question Becker's claim that allowing to die is far less injurious than direct, active killing to the dispositions of the conscientious health care professional. Would condemning John to a life of abject misery be less callous morally than the act of turning off his respirator?

A set of related questions arises over the administering of medication which hastens death. Was it reasonable for John's doctors to refuse to administer such medication, given that they had, in effect, already chosen to accept his death? Did they view the (active) withdrawal of life-support as nothing more than a passive surrender to the forces of death, and the administration of life-shortening medication as active conspiracy with the enemy? If so, is this view rationally and morally defensible? Is turning off a respirator in reality any more an act of killing than not taking steps to resuscitate Mrs. Jones? And even if it is, does the active/passive distinction have any moral relevance here? Or is it on a par with the view which allows a baby to wither away to nothing but prohibits active intervention to bring about its painless and speedy death?

Notes

1   See Mary Anne Warren, "The Moral and Legal Status of Abortion," in J. E. Thomas (ed.), *Medical Ethics and Human Life* (Toronto: Samuel Stevens, 1983), 99-106. See also Joseph Fletcher, "Indicators of Humanhood," *Hastings Center Reports* (vol. 12, No. 5, 1972).

2   See Paul Ramsey, *Ethics at the Edges of Life* (New Haven: Yale University Press, 1978), Ch. 4, 7.

3   See James Rachels, "Active and Passive Euthanasia," in Thomas, 291-6.

4   Lawrence Becker, "Killing and Giving Up," in Natalie Abrams and Michael Buckner (eds.), *Medical Ethics: A Clinical Textbook and Reference for the Health Care Professions* (Cambridge, Mass: MIT Press, 1983), 43.

5   Rachels, 292.

6   Rachels.

Case 8:3 Sue Rodriguez: "Please Help Me to Die"

Sue Rodriguez was a Canadian with Amyotrophic Lateral Sclerosis (ALS) or Lou Gehrig's Disease. She contracted the disease in 1991 at the age of forty, and by 1993 she was thought to have a remaining life expectancy of anywhere from two to fourteen months. The prognosis was that she would soon lose the ability to swallow, speak, walk, and move about without assistance. Eventually, she would lose the capacity to breath on her own without the help of a respirator.

In the early stages of her illness, Rodriguez decided that she wished to continue living so long as she had the capacity to enjoy life. Once she began to experience deterioration of her abilities, Rodriguez entertained the possibility of suicide. She wished to maintain control over how and when she died, and to spare herself the experiences she was destined to have once her illness reached its final stages. The dilemma she faced was that "by the time she no longer [was] able to enjoy life, she [would] be physically unable to terminate her life without assistance."[1] In light of this, Rodriguez petitioned the courts for an order "which [would] allow a medical practitioner to set up technological means by which she might, by her own hand, at the time of her choosing, end her life."[2]

Rodriguez's application was made to the Supreme Court of British Columbia which was asked to rule that Section 241(b) of the Canadian Criminal Code, R.S.C., 1985, c. C-46 be declared invalid on the ground that it violates Sections 7, 12 and 15(1) of the Canadian Charter of Rights and Freedoms. The relevant provision of the Criminal Code is as follows:

> 241. Every one who
>   (a) counsels a person to commit suicide, or
>   (b) aids or abets a person to commit suicide,
> whether suicide ensues or not, is guilty of an indictable offence and liable to imprisonment for a term not exceeding fourteen years.

The relevant sections of the Charter of Rights and Freedoms are as follows:

> 7.   Everyone has the right to life, liberty, and security of the person and the right not to be deprived thereof except in accor-

dance with the principles of fundamental justice.

12. Everyone has the right not to be subjected to any cruel and unusual treatment or punishment.

15. (1) Every individual is equal before and under the law and has the right to the equal protection and equal benefit of the law without discrimination and, in particular, without discrimination based on race, national, or ethnic origin, colour, religion, sex, age, or mental or physical disability.

Rodriguez claimed that, because suicide is not itself a criminal offence, *assisted* suicide should be legal. That it is not legal discriminates against those who are dying but physically unable to commit suicide without assistance. It also denies such individuals equal protection and benefit of the law. Rodriguez's claim was rejected by both the Supreme Courts of British Columbia and of Canada. In each instance, the majority of judges held that Section 241 reflected a legitimate state interest in protecting the vulnerable and was consistent with a widespread social consensus that human life must be respected and that institutions designed to protect it must not be undermined. According to (the late) Justice Sopinka, Section 241 "reflects the state's policy that human life should not be depreciated by allowing life to be taken."[3] According to the courts, any violations to Rodriguez's rights under Sections 7, 12 and 15 (1) of the Canadian Charter were justifiable according to Section 1 which reads as follows:

1. The Canadian Charter of Rights and Freedoms guarantees the rights and freedoms set out in it subject only to such reasonable limits prescribed by law as can be demonstrably justified in a free and democratic society.

A legal prohibition against physician-assisted suicide represents such a reasonable limit.

Shortly after the Supreme Court of Canada issued its ruling, Sue Rodriguez took her own life with the assistance of an unidentified physician, and in the presence of her friend and advocate, MP Svend Robinson. Neither Mr. Robinson nor the physician was charged under Section 241.

Case Discussion

(1) The Legal Landscape

In light of the Rodriguez decision, it is clear that physician assisted suicide is presently illegal in Canada. Such conduct violates Section 241 of the Criminal Code which makes it a punishable offence either to assist a person to commit suicide, or to counsel a person to do so. In December of 1995, a Nova Scotia woman became the first Canadian convicted of aiding and abetting a suicide after she helped a friend kill herself. The woman was given a suspended sentence. At the time of this writing, it is unknown whether a similar fate will befall Dr. Maurice Genereux, a Toronto AIDS doctor who pleaded guilty to two counts of assisting suicide. An Ontario court judge will pass sentence in March 1998. Dr. Genereux admitted to administering two potentially lethal doses of sleeping pills to two HIV-positive men, only one of whom died. Genereux reportedly prescribed 50 100-milligram capsules of Seconal to the deceased patient, Aaron McGinn, who reportedly "didn't want to suffer any more...[but] wanted to die with dignity."[4]

On September 22, 1996, an Australian cancer patient became the first person in the world to receive the assistance of a physician in committing suicide under legislation specifically sanctioning such assistance.[5] Since 1960, a series of judicial decisions in the Netherlands has made physician-assisted suicide and euthanasia legally permissible under strict guidelines. In the United States, two Federal Courts of Appeal recently ruled that there is a constitutionally protected right to choose the time and manner of one's own death. The Ninth and Second Circuit Courts of Appeal ruled in the spring of 1996 that Washington and New York state laws that prohibit assisted suicide are unconstitutional as applied to doctors and dying patients.[6] At the time of this writing, the Supreme Court of the United States has yet to decide whether to allow these two decisions to stand. If it does, then "physicians in 12 states, which include about half the population of the United States, would be allowed to provide the means for terminally ill patients to take their own lives, and the remaining states would rapidly follow. Not since *Roe v. Wade* has a Supreme Court decision been so fateful."[7]

(2) The Moral Issues

Many of the moral issues arising in the Rodriguez case are identical to those we examined in the preceding two cases. This is especially true of John's case (Case 8:2) where a fully competent individual asked to have his life terminated. Those who espouse the Sanctity of Life Principle will continue to insist that Ms. Rodriguez's request may not be honoured, despite the consequences of strict adherence to that principle. Those who see the value of human life to lie in what we can do with it, in what we can experience and the relationships into which we can enter while living it, will accept the possibility that the quality of Sue Rodriguez's life was such as to warrant honouring her request. Respect for her autonomy may require nothing less.

Despite their striking similarities, there are two principal factors distinguishing John from Sue Rodriguez. First, there is the issue of the dying versus the non-dying. As we saw, John was not dying, miserable though his existence no doubt was. It is difficult to take steps which one knows will result in the death of a person who is not dying and who may have years yet to live. But do this we must (sometimes) if we are to respect a patient's right to refuse medical treatment. To impose unwanted treatment on a competent patient is to commit a battery against him, something which is condemned in both law and morals. Sue Rodriguez, on the other hand, was clearly dying, though her death was not imminent. If we believe that there is a relevant difference between taking deliberate steps to *hasten* the dying process, on the one hand, (Sue's case) and taking deliberate steps to *initiate* a dying process on the other, (John's case) then in this respect it may be easier to justify helping Sue Rodriguez than it was to justify turning off John's respirator. If, on the other hand, one sees no moral relevance in the sheer fact that someone is already dying, then it will be no easier to justify honouring Sue's request than it was to comply with John's.

A second crucial difference between John and Sue Rodriguez is that the latter asked for active intervention aimed at deliberately ending her life, whereas John asked that active intervention aimed at preserving his life be stopped. Once again we encounter thorny issues surrounding the active/passive distinction. Is there, in the end, a morally significant difference between: (a) shutting off a respirator, with full knowledge that death will ensue, and with the intention that this should come about; and (b) administering a drug, or undertaking some other active intervention, with this very same intention? Those who think there is a difference often express it by saying that in the first case we simply "allow nature to take its course," whereas in the second case, *we* are the ones who participate in setting the course to the desired death. Whether we accept this account will largely determine how we respond to Sue Rodriguez's request. If we accept it, then we may be inclined to draw the line at (actively) assisting someone to kill herself. If, on the other hand, we insist that choosing to withhold active intervention when one knows that such intervention would result in continued life is as much an act of choosing as administering a lethal drug, we will be more inclined to accede to Sue Rodriguez's request.

Those who are morally opposed to physician-assisted suicide cite additional reasons for their position.

(a) Physician-assisted suicide is unnecessary. The suffering of dying patients can always be relieved through proper pain-management and palliative care.

There is no doubt that pain can often be managed, and dying patients can often be made comfortable. But sometimes this can be achieved only at the expense of full cognitive awareness. The loss of their cognitive faculties is something which many people dread, as an affront to their human dignity. As a result, they will prefer death over heavy sedation. If we are to honour their autonomy, should we not honour this preference?

(b) Permitting physician-assisted suicide will result in diminished efforts to improve palliative care.

It is difficult to see the force of this argument. It is doubtful that many individuals would likely follow in Sue Rodriguez's footsteps and ask for help to kill themselves. But regardless of how many choose that option, there will continue to be those who do not. There will therefore continue to be an urgent need to improve the situation of those dying patients who prefer sustained existence with appropriate palliative care. As Marcia Angell notes, "Good comfort care and the availability of physician-assisted suicide are no more mutually exclusive than good cardiologic care and the availability of heart transplantation."[8]

(c) Physician-assisted suicide is unnecessary. Individuals can always find the means to kill themselves without a doctor's assistance.
In response to this particular argument, Angell offers the following observations, which are worth quoting in full.[9]

> This is perhaps the cruellest of the arguments against physician-assisted suicide. Many patients at the end of life are, in fact, physically unable to commit suicide on their own.[10] Others lack the resources to do so. It has sometimes been suggested that they can simply stop eating and drinking and kill themselves that way. Although this method has been described as peaceful under certain conditions,[11] no one should count on that. The fact is that this argument leaves most patients to their suffering. Some, usually men, manage to commit suicide using violent methods. Percy Bridgman, a Nobel laureate in physics who in 1961 shot himself rather than die of metatastic cancer said in his suicide note, "It is not decent for Society to make a man do this to himself."[12]

Noting the fear of some dying patients that they will reach a stage where suicide is impossible without assistance, Angell goes on to make an additional point.

> If patients have access to drugs they can take when they choose, they will not feel they must commit suicide early, while they are still able to do it on their own. They would probably live longer and certainly more peacefully, and they might not even use the drugs.[13]

(d) Physician-assisted suicide is a form of killing, which is inconsistent with a physician's duty never to harm a patient.
While it is true that physician-assisted suicide involves killing, it is not the doctor who does the killing. Rather he or she facilitates the patient's suicide. Nevertheless, it might be argued that the physician *participates* in the killing, and that this participation is as inconsistent with the duty not to harm patients as would be the administering of a lethal injection.

In response to this argument, one might question whether facilitating the death of Sue Rodriguez would really have been of harm to her. She had reached a point where continued existence was no longer valuable to her, where the quality of life she had once enjoyed had been eliminated by her illness. In such circumstances, would the ending of her existence actually constitute a harm? And even if it would, would it not in fact be *less* harmful than forcing her to continue to exist against her wishes? Perhaps we should once again agree with Angell that the "greatest harm we can do is to consign a desperate patient to unbearable suffering – or force the patient to seek out a stranger like Dr. Kevorkian."[14] In some instances, it may well be that serving the best interests of a patient requires that a physician help her to end her life.

(e) Permitting physician-assisted suicide would put us on the slope to involuntary euthanasia.

As noted in earlier cases, slippery slope arguments rely on two principal claims. First, that the state to which we may slide is morally undesirable, and second, that the slide is inevitable or probable. Let us assume that involuntary euthanasia – i.e., bringing about the death of a patient against that patient's wishes – is clearly immoral and ought never to be legalized. The remaining question is whether physician-assisted suicide will inevitably or probably lead to this intolerable situation. If proper guidelines are observed it is difficult to see why the slide is inevitable. For one thing, physician-assisted suicide is not properly viewed as a form of euthanasia. In the latter case, someone other than the patient actually brings about the death, whereas in the former case, it is the patient herself who brings this about. That it is the patient herself who actually does the killing is perhaps the strongest safeguard against the slippery slope.

But of course, actions can be coerced, and so we must entertain the possibility that, once physician-assisted suicide becomes accepted practice, vulnerable patients will be pressured into killing themselves. The fear is that such pressure will result in involuntary acts of physician-assisted suicide. The pressure can come from two sources: others, who may stand to benefit from the patient's death, or the patient herself. In the former instance, family members who may stand to gain financially, or who find it emotionally draining or time-consuming to watch the patient slowly die, may exert subtle pressures on the patient to end it all sooner rather than later. In the latter instance, the patient may fear that she is burdening her loved ones, and may well consider herself under a Rossian obligation of beneficence or nonmaleficence to end her life.

The risk of abuse exists. But we must ask ourselves whether and how these risks can be minimized, and whether, once they are minimized, they are worth running for the sake of the competing values: i.e., honouring the autonomy rights and human dignity of patients like Sue Rodriguez. We are prepared to live with the risk that some people are being pressured into refusing life-sustaining medical treatment. Why should we not be prepared to live with the same risk when what is requested is assistance rather than withdrawal or refusal of treatment? Can we not build in the very same safeguards? If we do, there is reason to believe that the slide to involuntary euthanasia will not occur, as evidenced by reports from the Netherlands, where physician-assisted suicide has been practised for many years.[15]

Notes

1 *Sue Rodriguez v. The Attorney General of Canada and The Attorney General of British Columbia*, (1993) 3 SCR 519.
2 *Rodriguez.*
3 *Rodriguez.*
4 *Canadian Press*, December 23, 1997.
5 See Ryan C.J., Kaye M., "Euthanasia in Australia: the Northern Territory Rights of the Terminally Ill Act," *New England Journal of Medicine*, (1996) 326-8.
6 *Compassion in Dying v. Washington*, 79 F.3d 790 (9th Cir. 1996); *Quill v. Vacco*, 80 F.3d 716 (2d Cie. 1996).
7 Dr. Marcia Angell, "The Supreme Court and Physician-Assisted Suicide – The Ultimate Right," *The New England Journal of Medicine*, Volume 36#1 (January 2, 1997), 50.
8 Angell, 51.
9 Angell, 52-3.
10 Editor's note. This, it will be recalled, was one of the greatest fears of Sue Rodriguez.
11 J. Lynn and J.F. Childress, "Must Patients Always be Given Food and Water?," *Hastings Center Reports*, Vol. 13#5 (1983), 17-21.
12 S.B. Nuland, *How We Die* (New York: Alfred A. Knopf, 1994), 152.
13 Angell, 53.
14 Angell, 52. Dr. Kevorkian is the Michigan doctor who was tried several times for helping patients to kill themselves. To date, no jury has seen fit to convict Dr. Kevorkian, despite his open admission that he participates in physician-assisted suicide.
15 See, e.g., van der Maas, van der Wal, Haverkate, et.al., "Euthanasia,

Physician-Assisted Suicide, and Other Medical Practices Involving the End of Life in the Netherlands, 1990-1995," *New England Journal of Medicine*, Vol. 335#1 (1996), 699-705; and M. Angell, "Euthanasia in the Netherlands – Good News or Bad?," in *New England Journal of Medicine*, 676-8.

Case 8:4 Tracy and Robert Latimer: "It Was Right to Kill My Daughter"

On October 24, 1993, Robert Latimer deliberately ended the life of his 12-year-old daughter, Tracy, on his farm near Wilkie, Saskatchewan. Latimer freely admitted that he had put his daughter in the cab of his pickup truck and piped in exhaust fumes resulting in her death by carbon monoxide poisoning. Tracy had suffered from cerebral palsy and had been both physically and mentally disabled since the time of her birth. At the time of her death, Tracy weighed no more than 38 pounds. She had never been able to walk, sit up, talk, feed herself, or express her thoughts or wishes. She had suffered a great deal of pain throughout her life and had undergone numerous surgeries to correct orthopaedic and musculoskeletal difficulties. At the time of her death, Tracy was scheduled for further corrective surgery to relieve the pain of a displaced hip. She was not, however, in any mortal danger. Robert Latimer's defence was that his act was "mercy killing" and that he had acted only to relieve his daughter's continued and inevitable suffering.

On November 16, 1994, an eleven-member jury of the Saskatchewan Court of Queen's Bench found Robert Latimer guilty of second-degree murder. Judge Ross Wimmer sentenced Latimer to the minimum sentence required by law, life in prison (25 years) with the possibility of parole after ten years. Shortly thereafter, Latimer appealed the Court's decision and was released on bail. On July 18, 1995, the Saskatchewan Court of Appeal denied Latimer's appeal. Two of the three judges, Mr. Justice Calvin Tallis and Mr. Justice Nicholas Sherstobitoff, agreed with both the verdict and the sentence, arguing that these were necessary to protect the rights of the disabled. The third, Mr. Justice Edward Bayla, suggested in a dissenting opinion that the life sentence was too harsh for someone with Latimer's motivations. According to Bayla, the sentence imposed by law "exposes a stark inequality in the administration of justice in Canada in this sphere of wrongdoing." This sentiment, that the conviction was warranted but the sentence excessive, had been echoed in the media. Some drew a contrast between Latimer and Paul Bernardo, convicted in the sex slayings of teenagers Kristen French and Leslie Mahaffey.

Following his failure in the Saskatchewan Court of Appeal, Latimer appealed to the Supreme Court of Canada. On February 6,

1997, the Court ruled that Latimer's conviction should be set aside and they ordered a new trial. The Court had agreed that the Crown Attorney had committed an abuse of due process by requesting that the police canvass prospective jurors for their views on mercy killing.

On November 5, 1997, Robert Latimer was convicted once again of second-degree murder. The jury, though it found him guilty, recommended that he serve only one year in jail before parole. They had accepted Latimer's contention that the mandatory life sentence with no chance of parole for ten years amounted to "cruel and unusual punishment" and was therefore in violation of the Canadian Charter of Rights and Freedoms. In their view, Latimer was entitled to a "constitutional exemption" to the mandatory sentence. On December 1, 1997, the trial judge, Judge G.E. (Ted) Noble of the Saskatchewan Court of Queen's Bench agreed, and imposed a sentence of two years less a day. Mr. Latimer was to serve one year in prison plus one further year of house arrest. In issuing the exemption, Judge Noble noted that "If Mr. Latimer's situation does not warrant the granting of a constitutional exemption [to the mandatory sentence], then it is unlikely that any set of facts will ever arise where this rarely granted legal remedy can be made available to one who commits an act of compassionate homicide."[1]

Advocacy groups for the disabled were outraged by Judge Noble's sentence. Dr. Raffath Sayeed, president of the Canadian Association for Community Living, which lobbies on behalf of the mentally disabled, claimed to be "in shock."[2] Pat Danforth of the Council of Canadians with Disabilities, offered the following comment, "We're telling every senior citizen, every quadriplegic, anyone injured in a car accident that their life is of diminished value."[3] She further added, in response to the suggestion that Tracy's pain was unremitting and that her life was tragically debilitated, "Tracy's pain wasn't continuous. It was intermittent and situational."[4]

Before issuing Robert Latimer his constitutional exemption, Judge Noble provided an explanation of why he was prepared to take this highly unusual step. What follows is an excerpt from Judge Noble's reasons for judgment.[5]

As a person, Mr. Latimer is depicted as a responsible and hard-working farmer from the Wilkie area where he has lived his entire life. With his wife Laura they had four children, the oldest of which was Tracy, born with a very severe form of cerebral palsy which left her permanently incapacitated, and in order to sustain her life she required constant ongoing total care.

The evidence reveals the enormity of their task in caring for Tracy on a day-to-day basis, but establishes that Mr. Latimer shared in providing for her needs. Not only his wife but his sisters described his love and devotion to this child. When asked about the standard of care the Latimers provided Tracy, her doctor said "excellent."...

It is also clear from the ongoing history of this whole case that he is not a threat to society, nor does he require any rehabilitation. In summary, the evidence establishes he is a caring and responsible person and that his relationship with Tracy was that of a loving and protective parent. On the evidence it is difficult to believe that there is anything about Mr. Latimer that could be called sinister or malevolent or even unkind towards other people.

I move on to consider the gravity of the offence and the circumstances which led to the accused taking his daughter's life.

The gravity of murder need not be stated. It is recognized in our society as the most serious crime of all, and that is reflected in the penalty that has always been attached to its commission. Having said that, an act of murder like any other crime is committed in countless ways by people with countless reasons for doing it ... [The] law recognizes that the moral culpability or the moral blameworthiness of murder can vary from one convicted offender to another ...

From the moment [Mr. Latimer] was arrested, he told the police he did it because he wanted to put her out of her pain. The extent of the pain Tracy was suffering in the months leading up to October 12, 1993 is well documented by the evidence of her mother, the outside care-givers who attended on her, and Dr. [Anne] Dzus, the surgeon who had announced to Laura Latimer on October 12, 1993, that to alleviate Tracy's pain radical surgery to her right hip had to be done very soon. The extent of her concern is enhanced by her decision to move the surgery up to November 4.

We know Tracy had surgery before this to alleviate her condition. At four years they cut the muscles and tendons in her hips and she was left with a flail limb she could no longer control. While every effort was made to keep her muscles as flexible as possible, it must be remembered that Tracy, save for her head and one arm, was incapable of movement on her own, a fact which illustrates again the constant attention she required.

At age nine she required further cutting of her muscles and tendons to ease the pressure on her joints. This time she was placed in a case from chest to toes for a period of six months.

In 1992 her body had become so twisted out of shape that the surgeon placed steel rods in her back to straighten her body. After this surgery Tracy suffered severe pain because her right hip was dislocating regularly. This was thirteen months before she died.

By the time Dr. Dzus saw her on October 12, 1993, her pain was pretty well unremitting. All in all the evidence indicates that her health was slowly but steadily deteriorating. In the summer of 1993 she was in a respite home in Battleford, and while there lost several pounds by the time she came home.

When Laura Latimer told her husband on October 12 that Tracy needed more surgery to alleviate the right hip problem and that there was no guarantee it would stop the pain, and that Tracy faced further surgery as she got older just to alleviate her suffering, Robert Latimer took the decision to take the matter of Tracy's pain into his own hands. He considered a number of ways of putting her out of her misery, but finally settled on putting her to sleep with carbon-monoxide gas as the most gentle way of accomplishing his goal. We know that on Sunday, October 24, he carried out his plan.

Why did he do it? He consistently said his only concern was Tracy's ongoing pain and that he could not see any possible way she could ever be freed of the pain by the surgery which was scheduled to be done November 4, or that any future surgery designed to reduce her ongoing pain was anything more than pain management – certainly not a cure or anything close to it
…

The decision [Mr. Latimer] made was in clear conflict with the law and he knew it, but he did not seem to care so long as he accomplished his goal.

There are different ways of characterizing his decision to take Tracy's life. The Court of Appeal saw him as "assuming the role of a surrogate decision-maker" who then decided to terminate her life. I would characterize it by saying that he (and his wife) became the surrogates of Tracy at her birth and that twelve years later he decided, when faced with the despairing news that her pain would continue unremitting, that he must do his duty as her father to relieve her of that prospect. It is significant in my opinion that the jurors indicated through the questions submitted to the court that they too felt he should not have killed Tracy but they sympathized to a significant degree with why he had done it.

I repeat again that, in my opinion, the evidence does not in any way suggest he killed his daughter because she was so severely disabled. It is admittedly a difficult task to prove what motivates a person to carry out such a grave act as murder that was not somehow related to self-interest, malevolence, hate or violence. But in my view of the evidence presented in this case, which is for the most part clear and uncontradicted, we have that rare act of homicide that was committed for caring and altruistic reasons. That is why for want of a better term this is called compassionate homicide ...

[Would a life sentence without parole for ten years in this case] constitute cruel and unusual punishment? After much reflection I have concluded that the answer to that question is "yes."

Case Discussion

(1) Non-voluntary euthanasia

The primary moral issue arising in the Latimer case is whether it can *ever* be right deliberately to engage in non-voluntary euthanasia. It is usual in a case such as Tracy Latimer's to refer to "involuntary" euthanasia. The phrase "non-voluntary" is chosen instead to signal the fact that the question of voluntariness does not even arise in a case such as this. It is not as if Tracy was killed *against* her will. Given her severe mental disability, Tracy was never able to form and express wishes concerning her treatment that might be ignored or overridden by the decisions of others. As Judge Noble indicated, the Latimers assumed the role of surrogate at the moment of Tracy's birth, and for her entire life were faced with the prospect of deciding, not in terms of her expressed wishes, but in terms of her best interests. It was the surrogate judgment of Robert Latimer that those interests lay in termination of Tracy's life. In his judgment, it was not in the best interests of his daughter that she should live a life of unremitting pain.

Many advocacy groups for the disabled suggested that it was Tracy's disability which lay behind Robert Latimer's actions. Recall the words of Pat Danforth, "We're telling every senior citizen, every quadriplegic, anyone injured in a car accident that their life is of diminished value.... Tracy's pain wasn't continuous. It was intermittent and situational." Was this true, however? Judge Noble was clearly of the view that it was Tracy's unremitting pain, not her disability, that motivated Robert Latimer to end his daughter's life. But the question still remains: Were it not for Tracy's disabilities, would her father have contemplated ending her life? Is it possible that the only reason Tracy's pain was judged by Latimer to be sufficient reason for ending her life was that he judged the quality of her life to be so low as to be outweighed by her suffering? If so, and if his judgment might have been different had she not been disabled, or as disabled as she was, then perhaps the advocacy groups were correct. Perhaps we are on the way to eliminating disabled individuals whose lives are judged unworthy of continuing.

(2) The Slippery Slope once again

The Latimer case invokes fears of the slippery slope, whose logic, it will be recalled, is essentially as follows.

Assume we are now in State A. If we take a certain step and alter our attitudes, dispositions, practices or principles, we will land in State B. State B is desirable – or at the very least not undesirable. And so were we confident that we could remain in State B we would have no objection to taking the proposed step. But the slope is slippery, and so we are not confident that we could remain in State B. Any step towards B will inevitably or probably cause us to land in State C, which, unlike B, is undesirable. We have reason then, not to take the step towards B.

The slippery slope argument has, then, two pivotal claims:

i.   Movement to State B will inevitably or probably cause movement to State C.

and

ii. State C is undesirable.

Assuming that we do not wish morally to sanction the illegal actions of Robert Latimer, the question arises: Is this case evidence that our evolving attitudes towards practices such as the withdrawal of life-support, assisted suicide, and perhaps even voluntary euthanasia (State B), are leading us to the point where we will have no option but to accept the actions of the next Robert Latimer (State C)? Perhaps. As Aristotle might have said, once we disturb our disposition to fight death at all costs, it may become easier to sanction the actions of one who kills for compassionate reasons. But perhaps these fears are exaggerated. Virtually everyone sympathized with the situation in which Robert Latimer found himself. Many people believed that he did not warrant a sentence comparable to those often imposed on cold-blooded killers. But virtually no one thought that Latimer's actions could be fully excused, that he did the right thing in taking matters into his own hands in the way that he did. Virtually no one thought that it was his responsibility, as a father, to ease his daughter's suffering by eliminating her life. Is there room, in our moral thinking about these matters, for something analogous to the constitutional exemption which Noble was prepared to grant Robert Latimer? If we are not prepared to allow the kind of unregulated, non-voluntary euthanasia Robert Latimer felt compelled to pursue, should we nevertheless consider a scheme in which such actions could be undertaken by duly certified health-care professionals under carefully circumscribed and legislated controls? Or is this too far down the slippery slope?

In thinking through these questions, consider how you would answer were the facts slightly different. Suppose that Tracy had undergone the planned operation. Suppose further that during the course of the operation Tracy had arrested. Would the surgical team have been justified, under the circumstances, in not resuscitating her? Would non-action have been justifiable if the surgeon had sought and received, in advance, surrogate consent from Laura and Robert Latimer to a DNR (Do-Not-Resuscitate) order? If the answer is yes, then on what ground would you distinguish these particular steps from the ones taken by Robert Latimer? Would you once again be faced with the question whether there is a morally relevant distinction between active and passive measures resulting in death? Would it be a moral "cop-out" to sit back and let Tracy die on the operating table when you would not be prepared to take active steps to end her suffering?

(3) The Vulnerability of Tracy Latimer

Adding to the strong feelings of this case was Tracy's immense vulnerability. Tracy was a defenceless young girl with no capacity to decide or act on her own behalf. She had no capacity to speak for herself, or to prevent the actions of her father. We must, some argue, be ever vigilant that the interests of such vulnerable individuals are protected. This means that we must never sanction the actions of well-meaning persons like Robert Latimer, and never sanction a regulated scheme of non-voluntary euthanasia.

Does this argument have weight? Or does the vulnerability of Tracy Latimer point in the opposite direction? Robert Latimer clearly believed that, in light of his daughter's incapacity and consequent vulnerability, she needed to be protected from the suffering she was destined to endure. In his judgment, this vulnerability meant that he had no choice but to protect her from her incessant suffering by ending her life. Is his the better way of looking at the matter? Should we in this context accept Marcia Angell's claim that "The greatest harm we can do is to consign a desperate [individual] to unbearable suffering ..."[6]

Notes

1 As reported in *The Globe and Mail*, December 2, 1997, A8.
2 *Globe and Mail*.
3 *Globe and Mail*.
4 *Globe and Mail*.
5 *Globe and Mail*, A17.
6 Marcia Angell, "The Supreme Court and Physician-Assisted Suicide – The Ultimate Right," *New England Journal of Medicine*, vol. 336#1, 52.

Case 8:5 The Brain Dead As Teaching Materials

Sara Samuels, a 50-year-old corporate lawyer from London, Ontario, was admitted to the Emergency Ward of University Hospital complaining of severe dizziness and fatigue. Following an initial examination, Sara was taken to the ICU where she was placed on cardio-respiratory support machines. Approximately one hour afterwards Sara experienced a massive stroke and was declared brain-dead. Despite the death of her brain, Sara's heart continued to pump and her lungs continued to breathe, courtesy of the machines.

Tom Samuels, a chartered accountant, and their son Mark, a resident at London's Victoria Hospital, were promptly notified of the death and asked to meet with Dr. Julie Wallace, Director of Research Services at University Hospital.

Upon arrival at the hospital Mark and Tom were told by Dr. Wallace of the hospital's intention to use Sara's still functioning body for purposes of medical education. It was pointed out that the deceased had consented under Ontario's Human Tissue Gift Act to the use of her body for such purposes by signing the back of her driver's licence.

Mark and Tom were both surprised and greatly distressed by this revelation. Neither had been aware of Sara's action and neither was prepared to accept her decision. Tom's objections were those of a grieving husband who could not bear the thought of his loved one's body being probed and dissected, especially when it was still breathing and pumping blood. He was well aware, he said, of how medical research and education cannot proceed without the use of human bodies and of how very much more useful than cadavers still-functioning bodies can be. So while he agreed in principle with the idea, it was a different matter when it came to his wife's body. "I'm sorry," he said, "but I just can't bring myself to accept what you have in mind."

Mark's objections were a bit more complicated. Having once been a medical student himself, he said he was "all too aware of the indignities to which bodies are often subjected by callous medical students. Not for one moment am I going to allow that to happen to my mother." But Mark had other objections too. Unlike his father, who saw nothing in principle wrong with using brain-dead humans for purposes of medical education, Mark had moral reservations. "There has been much talk recently," he said, "of keeping bodies alive indefinitely for all sorts of macabre purposes. It's been suggested by some of my colleagues that the brain-dead could be 'harvested' of all things, for use in testing potentially lethal drugs or surgical procedures, or as sources of such things as blood or cartilage. To be sure, this will not happen to my mother, and it might be true that these sorts of things are not occurring anywhere at present. But it's only a matter of time – unless we now take a stand and insist that this otherwise inevitable and speedy progression to a brave new world be stopped. And that's just what I'm going to do. I won't allow you to take my mother's body. I insist that you turn off the machines and hand her over to us for proper burial."

Dr. Wallace was a bit dismayed by all this, and attempted to persuade Mark and Tom that their worries were unfounded. Sara's body would merely be used in teaching organ transplant techniques to student surgeons. The procedures would be well supervised and carried out with all due respect for the dignity of the deceased. The body would be returned within a week. Dr. Wallace's pleas fell on deaf ears. Tom kept repeating that he just could not bear the thought of his wife's "still beating heart being plucked and probed by the cold steel of the surgeon's scalpel." Mark, on the other hand, wasn't prepared to listen at all. "A matter of moral principle was at stake." Before the meeting adjourned, Dr. Wallace mentioned that the Human Tissue Gift Act legally entitles doctors to proceed on the basis of a duly signed driver's licence – with or without the consent of family members. She urged Mark and Tom to reconsider their objections, and to call her in the morning before any final decisions were made.

Case Discussion

(1) New Questions

Our ever-expanding powers to preserve human lives have brought in their wake a variety of moral dilemmas. Some of these were examined in the preceding three cases. Does a patient have a positive right to all available life-sustaining (or death-delaying) measures even at the expense of others who might benefit more from those very same resources? Should doctors take every step to preserve human existence, even when a patient judges his life to be of little or no value and requests its termination? Is it permissible actually to assist patients in achieving a "good death." These and other familiar questions concern the nature and value of human life and our duties to preserve and respect it.

But our new technologies also bring serious moral questions of a different kind. The very machines and techniques that enable us to save human lives also enable us often to save the human bodies in which (lost) human lives were once lodged. As a consequence, the bodies of brain-dead persons are becoming an increasingly valuable resource, one which many feel it would be foolish and perhaps even immoral to squander. This growing interest in the bodies of deceased persons is the pivot around which the various issues in the present case revolve.

(2) Ethics and Emotions

Tom Samuels is a grieving widower with an obviously very deep emotional attachment to the body of his wife. As with many who have lost loved ones, Tom finds it difficult to view his wife's remains objectively. This seems especially true given that her lungs are still breathing and her heart is still pumping blood. Intellectually he knows that she has gone but emotionally he can't accept it, despite Dr. Wallace's reassurance that Sara's body will be treated with all due respect. Tom is still incapable of assuming a "detached" perspective from which his wife's wishes and Dr. Wallace's intentions seem to make perfectly good sense. His emotions will not allow him to separate Sara from her bodily frame.[1] Would we want him to?

Tom's emotional attachment to Sara's remains is not at all uncommon. People often spend large sums of money to ensure that their loved ones "rest in peace and comfort." Appeals to the fact that lack of consciousness entails lack of pain and discomfort often fall on deaf ears. The emotional commitment to the body is far too great. It would be wrong, therefore, to ignore its impact in assessing Tom's reluctance.

It would also be wrong in other cases to ignore the similar feelings people have towards their own deaths and bodies. Many, like Tom, understand the strong humanitarian case for donation but still find it impossible to accept. Perhaps the explanation lies in an irrational tendency to project our conscious selves, with all our fears, concerns and feelings, into the death state. The prospect of being probed and dissected under such circumstances can be unsettling, to say the least.

Whatever the explanation, the feelings do exist and they are powerful ones.

It would therefore be a mistake to disregard feelings entirely in assessing other people's views on the donation of their bodies. But whether such irrational fears and concerns should be allowed to sway our moral decisions about our own bodies, or the bodies of loved ones, is a question which still needs to be addressed. Is it morally defensible to permit irrational fear and squeamishness to sway our moral judgments? Perhaps this is a morally biased way of describing things. What if, instead of irrational fears and squeamishness, we spoke of the emotional bonds between two individuals enmeshed in a loving and caring relationship, an immensely valuable relationship which is incompatible with the detached, rational perspective from which donation appears the only rational course. Must enlightened moral agents always be prepared, as Kant thought, to act in ways they find emotionally trying but which are nonetheless *judged* to be morally correct? Tom freely acknowledges the humanitarian benefits to which his wife's body can be put. There are many lives just as important to others as Sara's was to him that might be helped, even saved, by respecting her wishes. And Sara's wishes were clear. Respect for her autonomy would seem to require that those wishes be carried out. From both a utilitarian and a Kantian perspective, then, Tom's responsibility seems clear. But is it?

However we answer these hard questions, we are left with still further ones of no less importance and difficulty. If Tom's reaction is not atypical, then the question arises as to whether concerned parties, such as spouses and possibly even children and parents, should be consulted before we give our consent. Is Sara's decision properly viewed as a personal one where, as the "owner" of "personal property," (i.e., her body), she possessed a liberty-right to dispose of it as she saw fit? If the answer is no, and we wish to assign claim-rights to members of family, then how far should these rights extend and to whom? Should Sara have consulted her family, or perhaps only Tom, before she signed her driver's licence? Should she have at least informed them of her decision, to give them time to accept the idea?

If Sara was actually obliged to consult members of her family, then a further question arises. We know what the reactions of Tom and Mark would have been. Would Sara have been right to sign her licence under the circumstances even if she disagreed with Mark's moral stand and found Tom's reactions irrational? Even if she thought her moral duty was to benefit others by donating her body? But would she have had such a duty, given the reactions of her family? Mill instructs us to consider impartially the interests of all those affected by our choices and to choose the action which maximizes total happiness. Some people would no doubt benefit to an unknown degree from Sara's donation. But others (i.e., Mark and especially Tom) would most certainly suffer very great distress. Even if we must not allow our own irrational fears and concerns to influence our moral judgments, surely the fears and concerns of others, particularly those close to us, must play a central role in our moral calculations. It is far from clear, however, what decision would result from an impartial weighing of these competing interests. Is our sole duty to maximize, impartially, the happiness of all those affected by our decisions? If Ross and the feminists are right, and special relationships entail special duties and responsibilities, then is it not possible that Sara should have been more concerned with her family's feelings, irrational as they might have been, than with benefiting other people? Perhaps in this case a prima facie duty of non-maleficence towards her family, or the immense value of the relationships she shares with her family, would outweigh a competing duty of beneficence towards other people. So the question of what Sara's duty would have been had she consulted Mark and Tom is far from clear.

(3) The Slippery Slope

In addition to the emotional concerns he shared with his father, Mark had strong misgivings about the uses to which the bodies of brain-dead individuals can be put. His appeal was to the slippery slope argument which has been discussed in full above (case 8:4).

We are now presumably in the not undesirable position (State B) of allowing the bodies of brain-dead individuals to be used for purposes of transplantation, medical education, and research. To this, Mark appears to have no moral objection so long as the bodies are treated with respect. However, he sees an inevitable slide to the undesirable State C, about which he has grave concerns. This is the state described graphically by Willard Gaylin in his article "Harvesting the Dead."[2] Gaylin paints a disturbing picture of a world in which brain-dead "neomorts" are sustained and "harvested" for a variety of useful, humanitarian, purposes. As Gaylin notes, these neomorts "would be warm, respiring, pulsating, evacuating, and excreting bodies requiring nursing, dietary, and general grooming attention, and could probably be maintained so for a period of years."[3] We "could develop [bio-emporiums], banks, or farms of cadavers which require feeding and maintenance, in order to be harvested."[4] Uneasy medical students could practice routine physical examinations, including examinations of the retina, rectum, and vagina. "Both the student and his patient could be spared the pain, fumbling, and embarrassment of the 'first time.'"[5] Neomorts could also be used in the testing of drugs and experimental surgical procedures that "we now normally perform on prisoners, mentally retarded children, and volunteers."[6] They would offer a plentiful supply of transplant organs, blood platelets, skin, bone, corneas, cartilage, and possibly even antibodies. The possibilities are numerous and the potential benefits enormous. And yet, Gaylin writes,

> after all the benefits are outlined, with the lifesaving potential clear, the humanitarian purposes obvious, the technology ready, the motives pure, and the material costs justified – how are we to reconcile our emotions? Where in this debit-credit ledger of limbs and livers and kidneys and costs are we to weigh and enter the repugnance generated by the entire philanthropic endeavour?[7]

In attempting to explain our supposed repugnance, Gaylin cites William May, who writes, "While the body retains its recognizable form, even in death, it commands a certain respect. No longer a human presence, it still reminds us of that presence which once was utterly inseparable from it."[8] As noted above, it was undoubtedly the strong association between Sara and her body which was largely behind Tom's objections.

So we have here, once again, an appeal to emotional bonds (and perhaps the symbolic significance of the human body) over hard, "objective" assessments of costs and benefits. We also have, once again, a difficult question. Should any revulsion we might have towards Gaylin's brave new world – State C – outweigh, in our moral thinking, its considerable benefits? Gaylin notes that many who answer no will "interpret our revulsion at the thought of a bioemporium as a bias of our education and experience, just as earlier societies were probably revolted by the startling notion of abdominal surgery, which we now take for granted."[9] Still, he adds, there will be many who will answer yes, and defend their emotional response as "a quintessentially human factor whose removal would diminish us all, and extract a price we cannot anticipate in ways yet unknown and times not yet determined.... Sustaining life is an urgent argument for any measure, but not if that measure destroys those very qualities that make life worth sustaining."[10]

State C – indeed perhaps even State B – may also be morally problematic on other grounds. These are explored by Hans Jonas in his insightful critique of the Harvard Medical School's "brain-death" criterion.[11] Will our growing pragmatic interest in the bodies of brain-dead persons unduly motivate us to declare them dead? Once a person's death comes to be seen, not as the appropriate time for the death of his body, but as the appropriate time for that body to begin serving other useful functions, an individual's claim to his body is weakened. We may come to view him as a "temporary occupant," and as a consequence be too hasty in declaring him dead. To what extent should we follow Jonas in his concern for this possibility? Do his worries, together with those of Gaylin and May, provide sufficient reason to forego the useful purposes to which dead bodies can be put?

(4) Is the Slope Slippery?

We may, then, have reasons for thinking State C would be undesirable. But all of this is irrelevant for present purposes unless we have grounds for accepting the second pivotal claim in Mark's slippery slope argument – that movement to State B will inevitably or probably cause a slide to State C. Do we have sufficient reason to think that the donation of brain-dead bodies to medicine will probably lead to Gaylin's world? It is difficult to see why we should think so, but there are those who clearly do. Hans Jonas writes:

> Why turn the respirator off? Once we are assured that we are dealing with a cadaver, there are no logical reasons against (and strong pragmatic reasons for) going on with the artificial "animation" and keeping the "de-ceased's" body on call, as a bank for life-fresh organs, possibly also as a plant for manufacturing hormones or other biochemical compounds in demand.[12]

The "ruling pragmatism of our time," Jonas thinks, will mean an unavoidable slide to State C. "[N]o matter what particular use is or is not anticipated at the moment, or even anathematized – it would be naive to think [a] line can be drawn anywhere for such uses when strong enough interests urge them...."[13] Whether our pragmatism or our emotional and symbolic commitment to the human body would win the day is anybody's guess. To what extent we should be concerned to avoid the competition altogether is left to the reader's best judgment.

(5) Dr. Wallace

We now come to Dr. Wallace, in whom the law places the privilege of proceeding over the objections of Tom and Mark, who have no claim-rights against her in this matter. What should she do? Should she exercise her privilege? How should she weigh the family's concerns against the strong competing considerations? These include not only the potential benefits to others but also the important factor of Sara's autonomy. Whose wishes and/or interests should Dr. Wallace respect?

Some may be inclined to argue that the wishes of the living should always take precedence over those of the dead. "After all," it might be said, "What a person doesn't know can't hurt her; and the dead aren't capable of knowing anything." Tempting though this line of argument might be, we should pause to consider carefully its implications. Are we prepared, for example, to accept that wishes expressed in valid legal wills may be disregarded? If not, then why should we view Sara's wishes any differently? Consider also whether we really do believe that what one doesn't know can't be harmful. Would we view as morally acceptable and of no harm or consequence to the victim the slandering of a person who somehow never found out? Would we not think the victim wronged even though he never knew what was going on? If so, then should we not reject the claim that the dead, because they cannot know of it, cannot be harmed by failures to respect their wishes?[14]

How should Dr. Wallace respond to Mark's moral concerns and objections if she finds them groundless? Should they play any role in her deliberations at all? Consider that it would be Mark's mother's body being put to what he considers immoral purposes. Does this make a difference?

Finally, consider Dr. Wallace's response to Tom. She was no doubt correct to wait a day to allow him to become accustomed to the idea. Perhaps his emotional reluctance would subside with time. But if not, what should she do? Respect the autonomous wishes of the deceased and possibly benefit others – or respect the deep feelings of a grieving husband?

Notes

1   For arguments that the emotions underlying such inabilities are extremely valuable, see William May, "Attitudes Toward the Newly Dead," *Hastings Centre Studies* 1 (1972), 3-13.

2   *Harper's Magazine*, September 1974, 23-30.

3   *Harper's*, 26.

4   *Harper's*.

5   *Harper's*, 26-7.

6   *Harper's*, 27.

7   *Harper's*, 30.

8   *Harper's*.

9   *Harper's*.

10   *Harper's*.

11   Hans Jonas, "Against the Stream: Comments on the Definition and Redefinition of Death," in J. E. Thomas (ed.) *Medical Ethics and Human Life* (Toronto: Samuel Stevens, 1983).

12   Jonas, 310.

13   Jonas, 311.

14   On the conceptual difficulties we encounter when we speak of harming or wronging the dead, see Joel Feinberg, *Harm to Others: The Moral Limits of the Criminal Law* (Oxford: Oxford University Press, 1984); W. Waluchow, "Feinberg's Theory of 'Preposthumous' Harm," *Dialogue* XXV (1986), 727-34; and Ernest Partridge, "Posthumous Interests and Posthumous Respect," *Ethics* 91 (1981), 243-64.

Case 8:6 Religious Conflict Over a Life-Saving Blood Transfusion

Sally McCarthy was a normal, 15-year-old girl enroled in a local high school. For the past two years Sally had been a practising member of the Jehovah's Witnesses. When she was formally initiated into her local group two years ago, Sally solemnly declared her commitment to the sacred principles of the Jehovah's Witness faith. One such principle is that blood transfusions are a violation of God's law and are therefore prohibited under all circumstances, even life-threatening ones. Initiates into the Jehovah's Witnesses receive considerable instruction concerning the possible consequences of accepting the blood transfusion principle. They "go in with their eyes open."

At the time of her initiation, Sally's parents were both devout Witnesses. A year later, however, they became legally separated and Mrs. McCarthy renounced her faith. Mr. McCarthy continued to practise his religion in a nearby city, where he had moved following the separation. During the year following the split with his wife, Mr. McCarthy had seen Sally for only three short periods of time. Sally continued to live with her mother and her 18-year-old sister Jane. Joint custody of Sally was granted to the McCarthys by the court. Jane was never a member of the Jehovah's Witnesses, thinking their principles to be totally irrational. She is an avowed atheist.

Following the separation, Sally and Jane lived together peacefully with their mother, experiencing nothing more than the usual parent/teenager disputes. There were some rather hard feelings at the time of Mrs. McCarthy's renunciation, but these soon healed. Mother and daughter respect each other's religious freedom.

One Saturday afternoon Sally was involved in a very bad car accident. She was seriously injured and it was clear that she would die if surgery were not performed soon to repair the damage. Upon arrival at the hospital Sally was drifting in and out of consciousness. She could be heard to mutter repeatedly, "I don't want to die! Please help me!" Before the nature of her injuries and the consequent need for an operation could be communicated to her, Sally lapsed into a coma. On call that afternoon happened to be the McCarthy's family physician, Dr. Selby, who was given the task of asking for consent to surgery. Jane, Mrs. McCarthy, and finally Mr. McCarthy were summoned. Together they met with Dr. Selby in a counselling room at the hospital where the situation was explained to them. Without the operation, Sally would die. Upon questioning from Mr. McCarthy, Dr. Selby admitted that the surgery could not be performed without blood transfusions. Dr. Selby added that the surgical procedure required has a 90 per cent success rate with only a 5 per cent chance of paraplegia and another 5 per cent chance of death. He further declared that, from a strictly medical point of view, the operation was the only rational course to take. Finally, he offered the following comment, "Speaking in my capacity as a family friend, I strongly urge you to allow the operation to take place. Sally will die otherwise, something I'm sure none of us wants."

Mr. McCarthy objected that the operation could not take place if blood transfusions were to be involved. As an avowed Witness, Sally's clear wish, were she able to articulate it, would be that the operation not take place. Undergoing a blood transfusion would be, for her, an inexcusable violation of sacred principle.

At this point, Mrs. McCarthy became absolutely livid. She screamed at her husband, "You're a fine one to speak for our daughter. Where have you been the past year? Not in Hamilton at our daughter's side but off in another city. How dare you profess to speak for Sally and to decide what she would want? You hardly even know her any more! And we're talking here of Sally's life, not some foolhardy religious principle. Martyr yourself if you want; there's no way you're going to kill my daughter!"

As Dr. Selby looked on, dismayed by this shocking spectacle, Jane tried to introduce a measure of reasonableness into the situation. She claimed that, whatever the religious significance of Sally's commitment to the blood transfusion principle, it had no strict legal force whatsoever. Sally is, and was, a legal minor, who is incapable of providing valid consent or objection to treatment. That responsibility lies with her legal guardians, in this case, Mr. and Mrs. McCarthy. They must try to decide what is in Sally's best interests, not what she might wish. Jane added that it is questionable whether Sally's commitment to the blood transfusion principle could have been fully informed and voluntary anyway. Can a 13-year-old child fully appreciate the nature and consequences of such an act? If not, then it would be improper for the McCarthys to give weight to Sally's expressed wishes and beliefs. There is no option but for the McCarthys to heed Dr. Selby's suggestion and consent to the operation.

Mr. McCarthy again seized the opportunity to stress his daughter's genuine belief in the transfusion principle and the importance of her faith to her. "Just because the law treats her as an incompetent doesn't mean that we should. It doesn't mean that we should not respect her religious freedom, her right to decide for herself on such matters. Sally has the right to have her wishes respected, even though she is a minor and even though some of you find those wishes unacceptable."

Dr. Selby, as one might expect, was left in a state of perplexity and discomfort. On the one hand, there was good reason to think that Sally's wish would be to forego surgery, and to think that she had the right to have those wishes respected. On the other hand, there was some reason to question whether her formerly expressed wishes were fully informed and voluntary. There was also some doubt what Sally might actually say were she now able to express her wishes. In the light of this perplexity, Dr. Selby went before a judge to seek a legal resolution to this impasse. Imagine that you are that judge and that you are charged with the task of deciding whether the operation should proceed. What would be your decision?

Case Discussion

This case represents a tragic dilemma. Were Sally an adult whose previous – and continuing – commitment to the blood transfusion principle were clear, then the dilemma would not be quite so severe. It would, under such circumstances, be wrong, both morally and legally, to disregard her wishes completely because her religious tenets were viewed as silly but dangerous. Competent adults have the legal and moral right to refuse treatment, even for what some view as stupid reasons.

Of course, in some cases questions might be raised about the patient's continuing commitment to his or her religious principles. Consider Sally. If we were to assume that Sally was an adult whose consent to the transfusion principle was fully informed and voluntary at the time of her initiation, could we assume that she would continue to consent when faced with the inevitability of death? Recall her words upon arrival at the hospital, her pleas for help and her claim that she did not want to die. It is one thing to agree and commit oneself to an abstract principle in a ritual ceremony conducted among people whose acceptance one seeks; it is quite another to consent to the principle and its implications when one's very life is on the line.

On the other hand, we should take into account the following factors which seem to argue in favour of assuming Sally's continued commitment. Sally had ample time and opportunity to follow her mother's lead and renounce her faith. The fact that Sally did not do so, in the face of objections from both Jane and her mother, suggests strongly that her commitment was more than merely ceremonial; it was deep and abiding. As for Sally's utterances upon arrival at the hospital, one might question how much weight to place upon the disjointed mutterings of a frightened, possibly traumatized, accident victim. Do we have sufficient reason to infer that her plea for help was a request for whatever help could be provided – including blood transfusions? There is perhaps little reason to think that that possibility even entered her mind. As for her expressed desire not to die, perhaps we have no right to interpret this as indicating a desire to be saved at all costs. No doubt she wanted to be saved – but perhaps not at the expense of violating God's law.

So even if Sally were a fully competent adult, the court's decision would not be as easy as one might think. Were Sally an infant, on the other hand, the answer might also seem initially clear. It is one thing for an adult to decline life-saving treatment on religious grounds; it is quite another for an infant to be "sacrificed" on account of her parents' religious convictions. Children are not the property of parents, and it is always proper for the courts to intervene and act in a child's best interests if it is clear that those interests are not being served. In this case, the best interests of the child seem to lie in favour of an operation. But do they?

Seen through the eyes of an "average, prudent person," Sally's best interests clearly lie with the operation and the required transfusions. Seen through the eyes of an avowed Jehovah's Witness, however, those interests clearly lie elsewhere. According to Jehovah's Witness doctrine, transfusing an infant is the moral equivalent of child molestation. Transfusing an older child with awareness and acceptance of the transfusion principle is the moral equivalent of rape. A parent who therefore permits his child or infant to undergo a blood transfusion would be sanctioning a vicious violation of the person, thereby seriously compromising the child's best interests. Here, of course, the phrase "best interests" extends far beyond the child's interest in the preservation of her mortal body. Of greater interest is preservation of the child's soul. If this is so, then the question naturally arises, whose judgment concerning the child's best interests should hold sway with the Court? Mr. McCarthy's, or the judgment of Jane, Dr. Selby, Mrs. McCarthy, or the "average, prudent person"?

(2) The "Incompetency" of Minors

So far the discussion has assumed that Sally was either an infant or a legally competent adult. Of course she is neither and so the dilemmas posed are even greater. Sally lies in the troublesome grey area between infancy and adulthood. She is not legally competent to make decisions regarding medical treatment, but she may nevertheless be factually competent. She may, in fact if not in law, possess all the rational and emotional capacities of a mature adult. This fact about minors is given some recognition in law. It is a principle respected by most legal jurisdictions that the absence of legally recognized competency does not mean that a patient's wishes may safely be ignored. As Bernard Dickins notes,

> Even where retardates and minors lack capacity for autonomous medical consent, they may nevertheless have the power of con- clusive objection to treatment. Refusal of treatment should in principle be as informed as consent to it, but refusal based on emotional or irrational grounds may have to be respected. Further, age alone does not place the physical integrity of a young person under the absolute medical control of a parent.[1]

If Dickins is correct, then Sally has the legal, and no doubt the moral, right that her informed wishes be respected. This despite the fact that she is legally a minor, and even though an average, prudent person would agree to a transfusion. But now we return to the ques- tion addressed earlier concerning Sally's true commitment to that principle. Was her act of commitment fully informed and voluntary and therefore genuine? On the one hand, we must give considerable weight to the fact that she was a normal, intelligent, relatively mature teenager with a mind of her own. This she demonstrated by main- taining her faith despite the objections of Jane and Mrs. McCarthy and the absence of her father. If so, then as Kant would have insisted, she is a person whose autonomy and dignity must be respected, even in the face of undesirable consequences for her and all those others who might suffer as a result of her decision.

On the other side of the coin, one might again question whether a 13-year-old really can appreciate fully the nature and consequences of a religious tenet like the transfusion principle. One might also ques- tion whether a child's ritual acceptance of her parents' faith can truly be freely given. Many children are profoundly influenced by the need to please, to be part of their parents' way of life, and later that of their friends. Acceptance is for them of crucial importance. If so, can we really assume that Sally's commitment was genuine? If not, we are back with an earlier question: whose judgment should hold sway? Sally's? Mrs. McCarthy's? Mr. McCarthy's? Dr. Selby's? Jane's? Or the judge's own view concerning what is reasonable and prudent in the circumstances? A good deal hinges on how we answer this question.

Note

1   Bernard Dickins, "The Role of the Family in Surrogate Medical Consent," in J.E. Thomas (ed.), *Medical Ethics and Human Life* (Toronto: Samuel Stevens, 1983), 92.

Chapter 9: Scarce Medical Resources

Case 9:1 Dialysis Machine Shortages: Who Shall Live?

Forty-four-year-old Janet Greene was separated from her husband, had two children, and was on welfare. She also had a serious drinking problem. A victim of a traffic accident, she was admitted to the intensive care unit in her hometown community hospital. On admission Janet was treated for multiple fractures and abdominal injuries. When she developed acute renal failure she was treated with peritoneal dialysis. As soon as she recovered sufficiently she was discharged. For three months she managed to cope at home, but with poor kidney function. When she suffered a second bout of acute kidney failure Janet was readmitted to the community hospital. Tests revealed high potassium levels in her blood. Her condition indicated the urgent need for dialysis. Indeed, her physician was so concerned about her condition that he sought to get her admitted to a hospital offering long-term dialysis.

Janet's physician sought admission at two geographically accessible tertiary care hospitals. Both reported that they did not have space for Janet. When her physician inquired whether there was a patient with a poorer prognosis than Janet who might be "bumped" in her favour, she was met with stiff resistance. Both hospitals had adopted a "first come, first served" policy. It was pointed out that this policy was not only fairer than any alternative, it also avoided engaging in difficult quality of life decisions.

Janet's physician remained unconvinced. She queried the soundness of a policy based on chance rather than on a sound medical-indications policy. Is a patient with greater promise of long-term benefits not more entitled to a scarce resource than someone with a poorer prognosis who just happens to be on the machine? Furthermore, she was convinced that the fact that Janet had two children should be factored into the final equation.

Whose position is more justifiable morally, the formulators of the hospitals' policy or Janet's family physician?

Case Discussion

(1) Micro-allocation versus Macro-allocation

The case of Janet Greene presents a difficult micro-allocative decision. Such decisions are to be distinguished from macro-allocative ones. Macro-allocative decisions are policy decisions about which programs and services should be offered in a context of scarcity. For example, a hospital administrator sometimes has to make the difficult decision of whether her institution can afford to maintain a bone marrow transplantation program as well as a kidney dialysis and renal transplantation program. In a financial crunch a hospital administrator might have to decide between phasing out one program in favour of another, or instituting cuts in both programs even at the expense of reduced efficiency and accessibility. The resolution of these problems takes place in the impersonal domain of policy rather than the personal environment of clinical decision-making. It is the fate of programs that is at stake in macro-allocative decision-making, not the fate of identifiable individual patients at the bedside as in micro-allocative decisions. Nevertheless, while the fate of individual patients is not directly at issue in macro-allocative decisions, those decisions do affect individual patients indirectly. Any board-room policy to ration a scarce resource ultimately results in denying patients access to that resource at the bedside. That observation provides a cue for introducing micro-allocative decisions. Micro-allocative decisions become acute once the demand for a particular resource exceeds the supply. Even if at the macro-allocative level administrators decide in favour of spending a percentage of the hospital budget on long term renal dialysis, that is by no means the end of the matter. It might turn out that there will be more patients than machines. The difficult question will then arise: "Who shall have the scarce resource when not all can?" That is the question to be faced in this case and one that has a direct bearing on the fate of Janet Greene. Furthermore, what makes the decision so difficult is that it is a life or death decision. To withhold long term dialysis in the present case is tantamount to signing Janet's death warrant.

(2) Two Levels of Micro-allocative Decision-Making

Because the stakes in allocating scarce medical resources are often so high, it is desirable that micro-allocation decisions be based on sound criteria rather than be made on an ad hoc basis. In response to the question "Who shall live when not all can live?" two levels of decision-making need to be distinguished, each with its own criteria.

(a) First level: Eligibility Criteria
Eligibility criteria are geared to selecting patients who are likely to benefit medically from a scarce resource. Nicholas Rescher[1] cites three criteria:

(i) the constituency factor.
Sometimes in Canada when the demand for a scarce resource exceeds the supply, patients in an outlying region may be denied access in favour of patients who reside in the city in which the hospital is located. In the United States there may be restrictions on patients from out of state, or patients who fail to meet residency requirements. Where relevant the constituency factor has to be considered in the final decision.

(ii) the progress of science factor.
Patients could be turned away in a micro-allocative crunch if their particular need for a resource failed to fit with the research interests of the hospital. This criterion is usually justified by appealing to the principle that research makes for more effective medical interventions and that we have an obligation to provide patients with more rather than less effective medicine.

(iii) the prospect of success factor
All other things being equal it would be irresponsible to offer a scarce medical resource to a patient who is not likely to benefit from it, or is likely only to derive marginal benefit from it.

(b) Second level: Selection Criteria

Even when the task of determining patient eligibility for a scarce resource is completed, difficult decisions as to who among the eligible patients gets the scarce resource if there are more patients than machines still have to be faced. What resources are there to help with such decisions? The following criteria figure prominently in the literature.

Criteria of Comparative Worth

(i) Family role factor.

It has been proposed that the family role factor be taken into account in allocating scarce resources at the bedside. On this criterion, a mother with children would be preferred to a person with no dependents.

(ii) Contributions to society.

This is a two-pronged criterion that includes prospective service to society. This poses problems since it appears to advocate allocating resources on the basis of an individual's value to society rather than on the basis of the individual's intrinsic worth. (See Baby Jesse's case above, 7:2.) The "contributions to society" criterion meshes better with a consequentialist than with a deontological ethical position. If one views individuals as intrinsically valuable, it could be argued that they should have access to scarce medical resources regardless of their prospective contributions to society.

Where future potential may not be significant, one envisages appeals to retrospective service to society. A supporter of Ross might insist that past services rendered by individuals have created a prima facie obligation of fidelity. In absence of a stronger intervening obligation, this prima facie obligation would convert to an actual obligation and tilt the decision in favour of permitting access to a scarce medical resource.

First come, first served

For those who believe with Kant that persons are intrinsically valuable, some other basis of resource allocation than criteria of comparative worth is called for. If all patients are intrinsically valuable then it could be argued that there is no good reason why one patient rather than another should get the scarce resource. The principle of "first come, first served" is consonant with such a view. The adoption of this principle implies that if a patient without dependents is already on a machine, or arrives at the hospital even minutes before a woman with children, that unattached individual is entitled to the scarce resource. Does that commend itself as a defensible principle? If so, does it admit of exceptions, or does it virtually enjoy the status of a moral absolute?

(3) From Theory to Practice

(a) Prospect of success factor

The "prospect of success factor" appears to be more directly relevant to this case than the other two criteria of eligibility. It would appear from the physician's assessment of Janet that she requires long-term dialysis. May we infer this from the physician's efforts to get her patient admitted to a tertiary care hospital and from her disagreement with the allocation policy (first come, first served) adopted by both institutions? What does this reveal about the physician's moral commitments? Could the (at least tacit) rejection of the first come, first served criterion be entertained by someone who believed persons to be intrinsically valuable? But even if one agrees that it could not and opted for the intrinsic value of persons, would that imply that such a view is morally superior to the one held by the physician, or just different? If the competing views are just different does that mean that we simply have two defensible views here? Or is this a case that demonstrates the moral superiority of a consequentialist or utilitarian view? Would a consequentialist not be likely to argue that the first come, first served criterion simply testifies to a failure of nerve? With all its weaknesses a position that appeals to criteria of comparative worth tackles rather than avoids the tough decisions. Which of these two contenders makes the most convincing pitch?

(b) Family role factor

Among the selection criteria, the family role factor appears to be particularly relevant to this case and certainly figures in the family physician's proposal to bump a patient already on the machine in favour of Janet Greene. So, both the prospects of success and the family role figure in the physician's plea to consider bumping another patient in favour of her patient. The question then arises as to whether the family role factor could ever function decisively in a case like this. Suppose, for the sake of argument, that Janet's prospects were not better than any other patient competing for the resource. Would it then be morally permissible to introduce the family role factor as a tie breaker? If the answer is "Yes," what does this reveal about our view of persons? May persons be sacrificed to maximize overall benefit? If the answer is "No," does this mean that we should give no thought to whether, for example, the patient already on the machine is sixty-three years old and has had a reasonably good life? Do those who have had a good life not have an obligation to make room for younger people, especially younger people with children? While a utilitarian might argue this way, perhaps "have an obligation" is too strong a claim. While it would be commendable if they were to stand aside, perhaps they do not have an obligation to do so. If so, then volunteering one's machine to benefit another would be a matter of *supererogation* rather than *obligation*. It then follows that the force of the family role factor would have to be determined by the patient rather than institutional policy makers. It would also follow that the family role factor should be restricted to competent, conscious patients. Is that acceptable or not? If not, what modifications to the criterion would you propose to protect incompetent patients from being "sacrificed" to the interests of others?

(c) Prospective service factor

For some, this criterion will not yield much clout in the present case. A 44-year-old woman on welfare, with two children and an alcohol problem does not, some will argue, hold much promise of being a contributor to society. If this is true – which must seriously be questioned – should that make a difference to whether a patient has access to a scarce resource? Perhaps here we must heed the feminists' insistence that the broader social context in which such decisions are made should be factored in. Can it possibly be right to deny a person medical care because of social factors which make it very difficult for her to be a "useful" member of society? Is the conception of "usefulness" at play here one which a morally enlightened society can accept as a proper basis for allocation decisions? Will such a conception invariably work against women? Will it invariably work against those to whom fate has dealt a bad hand? Will it make us stop and think about the people we wish *to be*?

(d) Retrospective service factor

Some may argue that there is little evidence that Janet Greene has contributed a great deal to society. But perhaps, morally, this is beside the point. Among the reasons for objecting to the "prospective service" criterion is that it could be construed as imposing a moral "means test" on a group of particularly vulnerable people. For the reasons cited above, we must question whether such a "means test" is a good thing to have.

(e) Lifestyle factor

This is a criterion not considered so far but one which is ostensibly compatible with a consequentialist view. Heavy drinking and healthy kidney function are incompatible bedmates. To what extent, if at all, should access to scarce resources be made contingent on patients' conformity to lifestyles which do not work against the prospect of successful treatment? Should we, for example, deny heart transplants to people who will continue to smoke and consume fatty foods? Should Janet be denied dialysis unless she promises to quit drinking alcohol? If so, how far along this road should we go in denying treatment options?

Note

1   Nicholas Rescher, "The Allocation of Exotic Lifesaving Therapy," *Ethics*, 79:3, April 1969, 173-86.

Case 9:2 Budget Cutting in Neonatology and Perinatology

At its inception the high-risk perinatal program at Trelawny Medical Centre in Metropolis, Ontario, undertook to serve that hospital, two other Obstetric Hospitals in the city in which Trelawny is located, and the local region which shall be designated Region C. This undertaking came about as the result of an agreement among the three hospitals in Metropolis to focus level III neonatal and perinatal care at Trelawny in an effort to avoid duplication of the costly aspects of neonatal intensive care. Since long-term tracheal intubation and assisted ventilation require expensive equipment and higher levels of staff performance, level III care, which required such equipment and expertise, was restricted to Trelawny. The other two hospitals in Metropolis confined their services to level II care. The agreement proved to be congenial to the provincial government, which thought it would provide a more effective, economical, and specialized health care when needed. The government made a commitment to fund the program through an increase to Trelawny's global budget. The provincial government also created four more regions with neonatal intensive care focused in designated tertiary care hospitals like Trelawny. Since there was no tertiary care unit in the northern region of the province the government made a further commitment to underwrite the cost of transporting patients to one or other of the five regional centres. As part of a working agreement, one or other of these centres was obliged to accept such patients subject to availability of space. In the 1960s, when this regional arrangement was first introduced, the chance of a patient being turned away for lack of space was extremely remote.

That picture has dramatically changed. During the past two years alone, increases in requests for admission at Trelawny have strained existing resources to the point where the Neonatal Unit has been unable to fulfil its regional obligations. While able to honour all requests for admission from the inborn obstetric unit at Trelawny Medical Centre and from the city hospitals in Metropolis, the neonatal unit has been forced to refuse a significant number of requests for admission from Region C. Of 214 requests for admission from outside the Metropolis area in 1987/88, 36 (17 per cent) were refused for lack of space and/or facilities. In 1988/89, 99 out of 263 requests were refused (38 per cent). The rate of refusals of requests from Region C has increased from approximately 12 per cent three years ago to approximately 46 per cent this past year. The fate of the infants refused admission is not known. Pressures on the unit have resulted in frequent closures that have not only compromised its regional mandate, but also impaired the functioning of the Perinatal Obstetric Unit whose activities are inextricably bound up with the Neonatal Unit. Once the Neonatal Unit is full, requests from the region to admit high-risk patients to the Perinatal Obstetric Unit are refused. When it is time for pregnant women to deliver it is imperative that they be assured of the back up services of the Neonatal Unit.

The current crisis in the Neonatal Unit was precipitated by increased demands for services and a decreased capacity to supply services due to financial constraints. Governmental cuts in health care funding have made it impossible for the unit to fulfil its regional mandate. To do that would require a 40 per cent increase in beds. Because funding is not forthcoming, the Neonatal Unit has been forced to close repeatedly at the cost of turning away patients from the region. In addition, internal budget-cutting at Trelawny aimed at reducing the hospital deficit has resulted in further cuts in services. Beds in the neonatal unit have had to be reduced a further 7 per cent.

In making this last decision the administrators at Trelawny found themselves between a rock and a hard place. They were faced with the following options: (i) to selectively phase out certain departments or programs; (ii) to reduce budgets of high cost programs like neonatology; or (iii) to initiate across-the-board percentage cuts. They opted for a combination of (ii) and (iii). The avoidance of (i) was defended on the grounds that if departments or programs were to be phased out, it would be extremely difficult, if not impossible, to reinstate them. Option (iii) was justified on the grounds that it would be less traumatic, at least in the short run, than phasing out programs entirely. It was acknowledged that implementing across-the-board budget cuts was a stopgap measure to buy time to explore a more rational approach for dealing with the problem of providing health-care in a context of scarcity. However, the administrators readily acknowledged that the ploy would not bear repetition without seriously jeopardizing the full range of programs considered essential to a full-service, teaching hospital. As we shall see later, option (ii) proved to be unacceptable to the neonatologists and perinatologists at Trelawny because of its focus on costs in abstraction from outcomes (more on this under Alternative 1 below).

The pediatricians and obstetricians were less than enamoured of the formula for resource allocation adopted by Trelawny's administrators. In their response they offered two matters for consideration: (1) that their program was cost-effective and that in times of financial constraint the hospital had a special obligation to favour cost-effective over non-cost-effective programs; (2) that this obligation was even more pressing when those cost-effective programs were not duplicated in the region.

The Ethical Question

Did the hospital administrators make the right decision internally by (a) opting for across-the-board percentage cuts in an attempt to distribute the benefits more equitably; and (b) targeting high cost programs? Or should they have applied the cost-effective criterion more rigorously and phased out programs less cost-effective, particularly those programs that were duplicated in other hospitals or could possibly be accommodated in other hospitals in Metropolis? How heavily should the fact that the neonatal-perinatal program did not duplicate services within the region be weighted?

Case Discussion

(1) Exploring the Alternatives

(a) Alternative 1: Maintain full regional status by phasing out cost-ineffective programs

Neonatologists at Trelawny were quick to point out that their program had wide recognition for cost effectiveness in the field of neonatal intensive care of low birth-weight infants. This evaluation indicated that neonatal intensive care compared favourably with other health care programs at Trelawny and elsewhere which have also been evaluated in cost-effective terms. It seemed unfair, therefore, for a cost-effective program to have to face cuts while the hospital continued to maintain programs that had not been evaluated in terms of cost-effectiveness. Simply to reduce budgets of so-called "high cost" programs was not viewed as sufficiently discriminating. The consideration of costs without reference to individual outcomes jeopardized the notion of "effectiveness" in "cost effective" in the evaluation of health care programs. One neonatologist appealed to two principles that he believed should guide a rational approach to budget cutting:

(1) Health care that has been evaluated as more cost-effective should be preferred to that which is known to be less so, or to that whose cost-effectiveness is unknown.
(2) Among the cost-effective programs, those which provide unique services to a defined population should be preferred to those which provide services which could be obtained at other hospitals in the region whose budgets permit them.

Since neonatal intensive care had been favourably evaluated in terms of cost effectiveness and was unique in being designated "the only level III unit in Region C," it could be argued that services of the neonatal unit should be preferentially supported, and not selectively targeted for reduction.

The counter argument from advocates of other programs appealed to long-range consequences. It might be premature to phase out other programs at a given point in time. After all, if neonatal intensive care of low birth-weight babies had been phased out in the late 1960s on the grounds of cost efficiency, the cost-effectiveness of the neonatology program would never have been achieved. So even if, in other disciplines, cost efficiency is slower in being realized, it is unreasonable to expect that improvements in mortality rates or reduction in morbidity rates should proceed at a uniform rate in all disciplines. And if so, it is unfair to penalize useful, perhaps even vital, programmes because they lag behind in terms of cost efficiency.

(b) Alternative 2: Maintain full regional status by refusing to treat the highest-risk low birth-weight infants

The proposal to desist from treating low birth-weight infants originates with the critics of neonatal care. The target group of these critics comprises those infants who weigh less than 1000g at birth (although a lower limit of 750g would likely gain wider acceptance). Certainly if it could be established that a significant number of neonates had been receiving "inappropriate" care, a possible area for economising might have been identified. Neonatologists, however, deny that the charge of inappropriate care can be made to stick if by "inappropriate care" is meant that improved mortality rates have been relentlessly pursued without regard for increased morbidity. Studies do not corroborate this pessimistic view. Rather, in recent years, the mortality rates have levelled off and the morbidity rates have declined. Increased survival, of course, accounts for the increased demands for beds in the neonatal unit. Viewed one way, the pressures on the neonatal unit are a function of its success story. It is not surprising that they should cry "foul" at being penalized financially for their successes.

This rejoinder notwithstanding, infants over 1000g do fare much better than those in the 500-999g group, and the pressures on the neonatal unit could be relieved, if not eliminated, even if treatment were only withheld from infants weighing 500-750g. If only five babies were denied treatment the savings to the annual hospital budget would be in the neighbourhood of half a million dollars. Withholding treatment from very low birth-weight infants is one possible, if morally questionable, solution to the problem. However, as we shall see later, such "goal-rational" proposals are much easier to formulate in abstraction than to implement in practice.

(c) Alternative 3: Maintain the quality of the existing program by giving preferential treatment to local patients

Essentially this was the option chosen reluctantly by the neonatologists and perinatologists at Trelawny in the wake of governmental and institutional economising. Such forced preferential treatment of local patients was viewed as less than ideal by the neonatologists and perinatologists at Trelawny. They acknowledged that preferential treatment of local patients amounted to the abandonment of regional status, and this could not be done without imposing severe hardship on patients outside of Metropolis. Abandonment would not have posed so serious a problem if hospitals in adjacent regional areas could have been counted on to pick up the slack. Unfortunately, they too were stretched beyond their limits. Consequently, patients in the outlying areas of all regions were in difficult straits not only because of Trelawny's retraction of services, but also because of the severe pressures on the other regional centres. Initially, it is tempting to accuse Trelawny and the other centres in the region of discrimination against extremely vulnerable patients by accident of geographical location. However, the matter is not that simple.

Before laying charges of discrimination, we must consider the rationale for Trelawny's preferential treatment. The rationale offered was that patients who have swiftest access to intensive neonatal care have the most favourable medical outcomes. It is important that this information be factored into the final ethical assessment of the alternatives now being considered. Whether a charge of discrimination on morally irrelevant grounds can, in the end, be made to stick is the question which remains. If we cannot help all who need our assistance, on what basis may we choose among the deserving candidates? Would it be permissible to cite the government as the true cause of any harm befalling a person outside the local area? After all, it was government funding cuts which put Trelawny in the dilemma in which they now find themselves. Or is this simply an unacceptable way of "passing the moral buck"?

(d) Alternative 4: Limit access on a "first come, first served" basis

One way of remedying this unfairness would be to facilitate equal opportunity to all patients in Region C, as well as Metropolis, to gain access to the program. This could possibly be achieved by adopting the principle of first come, first served. That would afford peripheral patients the same chance of admission to neonatal intensive care as other patients in Metropolis. While such egalitarianism has much to commend it when considered abstractly, it poses a problem in practice.

One obvious problem with Alternative 4 is that equal access regionally imposes serious burdens on patients in Metropolis. But is that so bad? At least on the principle of first come, first served patients in Region C would have the same chance at neonatal care as those in Metropolis. The regional character of the program could thus be preserved even if in somewhat diminished form. What could be fairer in times of budget cuts? The benefits and the burdens of the program would be borne by all patients throughout the region.

A second problem with this proposal is that equality of access cannot be negotiated in isolation from other factors. Consider the following scenario. A high-risk pregnant woman in the perinatal unit is due soon to deliver. But an emergency admission to the neonatal unit from the region takes the last bed. What shall be done for our high-risk patient when her time comes to deliver her child? Since the unit is full to overflowing, a transfer to an outlying centre must be negotiated at a time when all skilled personnel are already over-burdened. Furthermore, even if the transfer could be effected, this would place the patient at increased risk. In light of this factor one might question whether rationing services in the region on a first come, first served basis in order to preserve the regional status of the program is a rational way of handling the budget crisis? Or is the whole idea unthinkable? Is there not a tacit and non-negotiable commitment to provide ongoing neonatal care for women at risk who have been admitted to the perinatal unit? Surely a part of the rationale for the integration of perinatal and neonatal services is to ensure more effective care of women at risk of giving birth to low birth-weight infants.

If this line of reasoning is sound, one is faced with a serious question: Does equal access, with babies lost or impaired because of additional risks incurred in transfers, come at too high a price? In times of financial crisis, can a principle (first come, first served) that increases regional access to a scarce resource at the cost of putting in-house patients at increased risk of harm be consistently generalized? In a crunch, how does one balance such competing claims?

How are the advocates of equal access to neonatal intensive care likely to respond to these queries? They might well acknowledge that the consequences of equal access are sometimes regrettable but, nevertheless, go on to insist that it is the only rational and fair way of allocating resources in times of fiscal constraints. At least, on this option, it is possible to claim that patients are denied treatment by chance rather than by design. For those who favour "preferred access" to neonatal care the chance-design distinction leads to yet another challenge rather than to the termination of debate. For now the question arises whether favouring chance over design does not lead to a "scapegoat ethic" in which hard decisions are left to fate, the government, or anybody, rather than being squarely faced by care-givers.

(2) Government Funding of Health Care

A position paper circulated by the neonatologists and perinatologists at Trelawny made the following terse observation: "Neonatal intensive care has been well evaluated, and compared to other forms of health care is among the most cost-effective. Our order of priority must be to assess effectiveness and need first, and the expenditure second." While understanding the context of caring from which this observation comes, it is not unproblematic. Even if effectiveness and needs are assessed first, in times of financial constraints there may not be sufficient funds to sustain existing programs, let alone to expand them. For the observation to have compelling force one would have to assume unlimited financial resources. In the 1960s the sky appeared to be the limit in the funding of medical research and medical programs. But as health care costs continue to escalate exponentially and all attempts at cost-containment fail, it appears we are now in an era of enforced constraints.

It should be made clear that these escalating costs are not necessarily the result of bad management. Rather the escalating costs are due, in no small measure, to the successes or partial successes of medicine. This is particularly true of neonatal intensive care. Success in saving low birth-weight babies accounts for increasing acuity in patient illness. The greater the number of survivors, the greater the demands for more sophisticated forms of ongoing care.

Nor is the reference to "needs" unproblematic. Yesterday's wants translate swiftly into today's needs. Neither is the cost-effectiveness criterion for allocating scarce medical resources trouble-free. If one makes rigorous cost-effective interdisciplinary comparisons, doubtless one could phase out programs and do so with remarkable and commendable efficiency and consistency. The only trouble is that many sufferers would be denied treatment. But is that so serious a consequence? Is no treatment not worse than cost-ineffective treatment? An unequivocal affirmative answer to that question may be overly simplistic. The notion of "cost-benefit" as well as "cost-effectiveness" must be factored into the final equation. At least as long as beneficial cost-ineffective programs are in operation, not only do patients benefit, but there is always a chance that those programs can be made more cost-efficient. If such programs are phased out, the benefits to patients as well as the opportunity to improve the cost-efficiency will both be lost. So while there may be a disparity between cost-benefit and cost-effectiveness in comparing programs, it is not self-evident that programs should be phased out solely on cost-effective criteria.

But that is not all. When administrators and care-givers are confronted with a budget crisis, what is practically feasible must be realistically assessed. It is notoriously difficult to phase out departments or programs. While there is a need for more rigorous comparative figures on the cost-effectiveness of programs, the implementation of the results will still be extremely difficult. It is easier for humans to approximate hyper-rational, Vulcan thinking than actually to engage in Vulcan behaviour. While Mr. Spock (the Star Trek character) might have had no difficulty in harmonizing his behaviour with his logical assessments, human beings often find themselves caught in the crossfire between the dictates of reason and the tug of compassion. And this is not necessarily a bad thing, as Captain Kirk and Dr. McCoy repeatedly reminded Spock. So while it may be true that in cost-effective programs more patients will benefit for less financial outlay, may it not be preferable meanwhile that some be helped rather than none?

(3) Goal- versus Value-Rational Choices

As difficult as cost-cutting is for administrators, many of whom are physicians themselves, it is nevertheless true that cost-cutting policies are formulated at some distance from the bedside. And this can make a difference. Administrative cost-cutting is done *in abstracto*. General policies operate at the statistical rather than the clinical level, with figures and not with actual patients. It is easier to engage in goal-rational thinking when dealing with figures rather than with actual sick patients. Hence the coining of aphorisms like "Don't think like a practitioner when making hospital policy." To this practitioners are likely to reply, "Don't expect us to think like policy-makers at the bedside." Practitioners' responses are frequently more likely to be value-rational rather than goal rational. They inquire, "How can a humane society let these patients die? Think of the message we shall send out to sufferers in our society if we let one of these infants die." So a split between setting limits to health care by policy-makers and the clamour for a greater share of resources by practitioners emerges. There is a part of practitioners that longs to be free from policy-making and cries out, "Set the limits for intervention and we will comply with them," and another part of them that expresses itself in patient advocacy. As patient advocates they will then push the system to its limits on behalf of those in need of medical care. So wherever the internal, institutional parameters are set, practitioners are likely to push the system to its limits, and even beyond its limits, on behalf of their patients. It is reasonable to ask whether we would want our health care practitioners to be able to act in any other way. Recall the lessons of Aristotle concerning the demands of virtue.

Away from the bedside, care-givers sometimes assert that health care cannot endure the split between policy-making and therapy. Somehow there has to be a feed-back loop from policy to practice and practice to policy lest patients become the victims of professional schizophrenia that oscillates between being policy-makers and being care-givers. Whether this is possible is a question which has yet to be answered.

Chapter 10: Organ and Tissue Donation

Case 10:1 Anencephalic Infants as Donors

In the thirtieth week of her pregnancy, Mrs. Annette Wingrove presented herself at Metropolis Medical Centre for routine ultrasound testing. The test revealed her to be carrying a fetus afflicted with anencephaly. Mrs. Wingrove's physician undertook to communicate the results of the test to Annette and her husband, Mervyn. On hearing the results of the test, both wife and husband were terribly distraught. The physician explained that their baby's brain had not developed normally. Ultrasound revealed that there was almost nothing beyond a brain stem. This meant that their child could not be expected to function at more than the level of some basic reflex activities like heartbeat and breathing. Furthermore, on the basis of best medical prognosis, their child would be born irreversibly dying. At most, they could not expect their child to live more than a few days.

Annette wrung her hands and inquired, "What are we to do?" Her physician answered, "I can only tell you what others have done in this situation; they have opted to terminate their pregnancy."

"But I don't believe in abortion," responded Annette.

"Neither do I in normal circumstances," chimed in her husband. "But the baby's irreversible condition makes a difference. Why should you have the added burden of carrying our child to term only to stand by and watch her die? [Ultrasound had revealed the sex of their anencephalic child] So, as hard as it is for both of us to contemplate an abortion, it may be more bearable than the alternative. But of course, if you prefer to carry our child to term, then I will be as supportive as I can."

Annette then recalled the case she had read of another woman in a similar predicament who had carried her anencephalic child to term and offered her child's organs for transplantation. In this way the woman had felt that her child's life and death were endowed with profound meaning. "Would something like that be possible for me and my child?" she inquired. "If so, it would help to assure me that my child's brief life had not been lived in vain."

The physician responded, "While we do not have the facilities to do paediatric organ transplantation at Metropolis Medical Centre, there is time to explore that option at a centre where they do."

At this point, obviously agitated, Annette's husband said, "I am not at all comfortable with that proposal. It's one thing to donate one's own organs for transplantation, quite another thing to volunteer someone else's organs. It may be true that our child will be born without higher brain function. But if we do decide to allow her to come to term, then we should offer her care and comfort in her dying rather than subject her to procedures to which she is unable to consent. It would be different if we were consenting to procedures (if there were any) that might be of potential benefit to her. It is quite another thing to consent to donating her organs to benefit others."

"But," Annette replied, "I would like to think that this harrowing experience could be given some meaning. Would you rather that our child's organs be wasted, when they might be used to benefit another child?"

To which her husband replied, "I can enter into your wish to invest this whole terrible experience with meaning. I would like that too. But meaning for whom? For our child or for us? I am sure it is something that might possibly make us feel better, but I don't see how it would benefit our child. I would prefer that our dying child be treated with dignity and be assured appropriate care while dying rather than subjected to the trauma of organ transplantation. After all, we are not just talking about a standard post mortem, but about taking organs from a child whose heart still beats and who still breathes. I just can't bear to think about it and I can't be a party to it."

Case Discussion

Ostensibly, Annette's outlook is more reasonable than her husband's. Who can deny that it is better to use their child's organs in an attempt to save the life of another child, rather than to allow those organs to disintegrate in a burial plot, or be incinerated at a crematorium? Since this child will be born irreversibly dying, her organs can be of no use to her. While it would be insensitive to express these points that bluntly in a counselling session, they appear to be the bottom line in any reasonable approach to this case.

Would that things were that simple. Mervyn's misgivings are also deep-seated. There is something repellant about using an extremely vulnerable and irreversibly dying infant as a mine of organs for possible transplantation. [Recall our discussion of a very similar point in Case 8:5 above.] Should not dying infants, as Mervyn proposes, be offered palliative care and treated with dignity until they die? This view is by no means idiosyncratic. It is shared by many physicians, health care professionals, and members of the general public.

In sorting out the differences between Annette's and Mervyn's viewpoints we need to consider several things.

(1) Modifying Brain Death Criteria

According to the definitions of brain death currently accepted in most, if not all, North American jurisdictions, anencephalic infants, while born dying, are not, "brain dead." But if they are born dying rather than brain dead then, strictly speaking, they are *not* candidates for organ donation. They would need to meet the criteria for brain death (particularly the inability to breathe on one's own) to be candidates for organ retrieval. Hence, at first glance, Annette's offer, while generous, is unacceptable. If there were not a pressing need for organs coupled with a serious shortage of them that would have been the end of the matter. The need and the shortage, however, have prompted calls for the formulation of a new definition of "brain death." A new definition would facilitate a reclassification of anencephalics as "brain dead" rather than dying and thus admit them to the pool of potential organ donors.

The question then arises whether this definitional manoeuvre is open to the same criticism as the one levelled by Hans Jonas at the original definition of "brain death," namely, that the need for organs introduces practical and extraneous considerations that compromise the theoretical purity of the definition.[1] Jonas argues that we should be clear about the definition of "brain death," independent of the benefits of organ donation to others. In the present context one might be tempted to ask a prior question, "Why do we need another definition of death?" Until now there have been no problems with determining the kind of care appropriate for anencephalic infants born dying. Why the urgency to reclassify the irreversibly dying as dead? Is it not that we need the organs? This was Jonas's worry about the original definition. Practical, and on his view extraneous, considerations dictate the definition of death; the anencephalic infant's *medical* condition does not. Furthermore, it is moot whether the redefinition will stop at anencephalics. What would prevent its gradual extension to sufferers from hydroencephaly and massive encephaloceles? [The meaning of these terms will be explained presently.] It appears that we are stepping onto a lexicographer's slippery slope unless a way can be found to find a foothold on the slope to prevent the slide beyond anencephalics. But even if a foothold can be cut on the slope and the definitional enterprise can be halted after accommodating anencephalics, this may not avoid Jonas's worry about compromising the theoretical purity of the definition of death. He might well still view it as an attempt to reclassify the dying as dead in order to harvest their organs.

Consider, now, whether the purity of definition Jonas appears to seek is possible. One might ask whether "death" is something which *can* be defined independently of practical, moral considerations. Perhaps the term "death" is as partly evaluative as terms like "promise," "obligation," and "virtue." If so, then perhaps we cannot even begin to define "death" without considering the moral questions Jonas appears to want us not to ask. If we cannot, then cases like the one currently under discussion appropriately prompt the partly moral questions of definition which we have hitherto ignored. We have ignored them because of our widespread agreement on the currently accepted definition of death which has, up till now, served us well. But new advances in medical technology disturb that agreement and therefore prompt the moral questions we now must ask.

(2) Anencephalics as a Unique Class of Patients

Suppose, all things considered, one is unwilling to redefine "death" so as to accommodate the measures being contemplated. An alternative to redefining "brain death" in a way consistent with using anencephalics as organ donors is to treat them as a unique class of patients. The uniqueness requirement would allow that anencephalics are dying rather than "brain dead," but then go on to restrict donations by the dying to anencephalics alone. The justification for this is that anencephalics are born irreversibly dying, and without the higher-level brain function necessary for consciousness. Certainly anencephaly gives several indications of being a carefully circumscribed malady. It is characterized by: (a) certainty of diagnosis. The criteria for anencephaly are clear; (b) certainty of prognosis. Anencephalics are imminently and irreversibly dying; (c) inaccessibility to active treatment; and (d) absence of higher-level brain function. What other category of sufferers meets these criteria? On the basis of these characteristics it would appear that a decision to use anencephalics as donors is self-insulating.

But uniqueness is not that easily circumscribed. For example, are hydrocephaly, massive encephaloceles, or severe brain damage due to inter-cranial bleeding so clearly distinguishable from anencephaly as to render the uniqueness claim plausible? In hydrocephaly the brain is lacking and the brain cavity is filled with fluid. An encephalocele is the brain analogue of a spina bifida and involves a protrusion of brain substance of varying degrees of severity. In massive inter-cranial bleeding, blood displaces brain tissue. All three conditions, if severe enough, share the criteria alleged to constitute the uniqueness of the anencephalic. Since this is so, it would appear to be unjust to harvest an anencephalic's organs while protecting hydrocephalics, sufferers from massive encephaloceles, and infants who have sustained massive brain haemorrhages. Would such disparity in treatment not be *discriminatory* since it would involve us in what Aristotle viewed as the essence of injustice: treating equals unequally? One could, of course, advocate yet another redefinition of "brain death" to take care of these other severely afflicted sufferers. But then perhaps we really are on a slippery slope. If so, then perhaps we are far better off facing the morally loaded questions of definition this manoeuvre was intended to avoid.

(3) Modifying the Treatment of One Patient to Benefit Others

The expression "benefit others" is ambiguous. It may refer to the physical benefit of the potential recipient of an anencephalic's organs or to the psychological benefit of organ donation to the parents for whom the tragedy may be invested with meaning. In either case the benefits accrue to others, not to the anencephalic child. If we are not careful, will we not end up treating anencephalics as a mere means to benefiting others? Whether the second formulation of Kant's

Categorical Imperative can get a grip on this case is debatable. The moral impropriety of treating individuals as means presupposes that they are ends in themselves, and it is questionable whether anencephalics have this moral status. For Kant at least, to qualify as ends in themselves, individuals have to be capable of moral agency. Anencephalics neither are, nor are capable of, ever being moral agents. Since this is so they do not fall directly under the protective umbrella of the Kantian principle. Does failure to come under the direct protection of the Categorical Imperative warrant the subjection of anencephalics to organ transplantation, experimentation, or any procedures whatsoever without moral qualms? Do we have obligations to our human offspring even if they fail to qualify as moral agents?

One possible way of dealing with this issue involves drawing a distinction between *moral agents* and *moral subjects*. While "normal" newborns are bearers of rights and require that surrogates act in ways consistent with the exercise of those rights, certain "abnormal" infants (and abnormal adults, for that matter) are arguably not bearers of rights at all. Nevertheless they may be moral subjects to whom we owe certain obligations. That is to say, certain obligations intervene between them and the uses to which we may be tempted to put them for the good of others. This suggestion will be explored further in the next section.

(4) Surrogate Consent and the Anencephalic Newborn

Suppose we agree that anencephalics are neither moral agents nor capable of moral agency, and also that they are born dying. Consider now whether a question posed by Henry K. Beecher could reasonably be extended from "unconscious patients" to anencephalics, "Can society afford to discard the tissues and organs of the hopelessly unconscious patient where they could be used to restore the otherwise hopelessly ill, but still salvageable individual?"[2]

Beecher's question occurs in the context of a perceived need for a definition of "brain death" in order to avoid "wasting" human organs that could be used to save the lives of others. Since the question is a rhetorical one, it betrays a commitment to beneficence as the overriding consideration. And why not, since patient autonomy and even the potentiality for it seem negated by absence of higher brain functioning? Any bow in the direction of patient autonomy will have to be made by a surrogate. Genuine surrogate consent seeks to implement the patient's previously expressed wishes where those wishes are known. Where those wishes have not been previously expressed (and in the case of anencephalics cannot be expressed), then surrogate consent should be exercised in a way that promotes the patient's best interests.

It is difficult, however, to determine what the anencephalic's best interests could be. Indeed, because anencephalics lack consciousness and have no desires, it is arguable that they have no interests whatsoever. But suppose that they do. Since anencephalics are born *dying*, one might concede that they are at the very least entitled to such palliative care as is consistent with making them "comfortable" while they undergo the dying process. (It is questionable, of course, whether a being which lacks consciousness is in a position to experience comfort or distress.) Although aggressive care is counter-indicated since it would involve throwing roadblocks in the way of the anencephalic's irreversible dying, offering whatever palliative care might seem appropriate would be consistent with honouring the obligations owed to moral subjects. But do we have further obligations beyond this? Do we have the right to subject anencephalic newborn infants to non-therapeutic procedures calculated only to benefit others (whether other patients' physical needs or the parents' psychological needs)? While it is morally licit to volunteer one's own organs for transplantation, whether at the time or by advance directives, do we have the right to volunteer our children's organs even though they may be irreversibly dying and lack the capacities necessary to be aware of what is happening to them?

(5) Needs and Entitlements

The need for organ transplantation of infants must be acknowledged. The question then arises: "Are we justified in moving from the need for organs to the right to take organs?" Certainly the language of "taking" jars our sensitivities. The legal limits of organ donation in the United States are set by the Uniform Gift Tissue Act (1986) with its emphasis on giving rather than taking. The same emphasis on giving pervades the Canadian Human Gift Tissue Act. Suffice it to say that the strength of one patient's need does not create an entitlement to another patient's organs. There is at present no movement toward a policy which would permit the *routine* retrieval of organs from anencephalics (or any of the other unfortunates mentioned above) for transplantation. Even the uniqueness proposal considered earlier incorporates parental consent as insurance against routine retrieval. Perhaps, though, the requirement of parental consent is merely a procedural ploy, one which is insufficiently protective of anencephalics (and others in comparable situations). Can a manoeuvre that addresses the question "Who decides when infants cannot?" address satisfactorily the substantive question "On what grounds shall such decisions be made?" What makes the decision whether to donate the organs of anencephalic infants so difficult is the tug between social gain (benefit to others) and patient inviolability. If the distinction between moral agents and moral subjects is sound, then there may be obligations owed to the anencephalic which may not be overridden by the needs of others, whether they be the need of parents to find meaning in tragedy or the need of a potential recipient for the anencephalic infant's organs. We might also give consideration to the *symbolic* significance and value of the anencephalic infant. [For fuller treatment of the symbolic significance of the body refer to Case 8:5.] An anencephalic infant is not simply a conglomeration of tissue to be harvested to benefit other sufferers: it is a human child, born without the capacities necessary for meaningful human life, but a child nonetheless. What effect will there be upon our moral *sensitivities* if we take this step? Once we begin to view anencephalic infants as a source of organs, are we on the road to viewing it as a conglomeration of tissues? And if we allow ourselves to view these unfortunate children in this way, are we on the road to so viewing other vulnerable individuals? Is the ability to view members of our human family in this way consistent with the virtuous dispositions Aristotle thought essential to moral life? If we say no, are we merely allowing squeamishness and irrational emotion to stand in the way of moral progress?

Taking the above into account, now ask yourself the following question: "Should a dying anencephalic infant be given the same consideration and care as any other dying patient?"

Notes

1 Hans Jonas, "Against the Stream: Comments on the Redefinition of Death" in John E. Thomas (ed.), *Medical Ethics and Human Life* (Toronto: Samuel Stevens, 1983), 307.

2 Jonas.

Case 10:2 Fetal Tissue Transplantation

January 4, 1998

Dr. Cesar Manuel
Hospital Salvador Mario

Dear Dr. Manuel,

I have read of your pioneer work in the treatment of Parkinson's disease and am writing to you to explore the possibility of having my father admitted to your hospital for treatment.

My father has Parkinson's disease and has been treated with Sinemet (Levidopa-Carbidopa). His tolerance of the drug has been poor. His movements have become markedly more spastic and he has a severe case of hemolytic anaemia. I broached the possibility of a fetal transplant with the specialists at Xville Medical Centre, only to learn that up to the present time experiments with fetal materials have been restricted to animal studies. There is no immediate prospect of a shift from animal to human subjects.

The possibility of autografting [the grafting of his own tissue] has been seriously considered but because of my father's age (he is 69) it is feared that he would not survive the surgery. I understand that this may be due to the fact that autografting involves a double dose of surgery: laparotomy to retrieve his own bodily tissue for transplant, and craniotomy to implant this tissue in the brain.

I have been informed that you and your team at Hospital Salvador Mario have experimented with fetal tissue transplants for Parkinson's disease with an encouraging degree of success and with no adverse side effects reported to date.

I am at present in the eighth week of pregnancy and am prepared to seek a therapeutic abortion at the critical time to make fetal tissue available for transplantation to help alleviate my father's suffering. Over the years he has made tremendous sacrifices for his family, and especially for me his youngest child. You might say that I am the beneficiary of his sacrificial love and devotion and owe him a particular debt of gratitude. While I can have another child later, my father's needs are urgent and immediate. I assure you that I have thought through this matter carefully and have weighed the pros and cons. While I feel regret at the prospect of an abortion, I feel a greater obligation to do whatever I possibly can to alleviate my father's suffering. He would do the same for me if he were able and our fortunes were reversed. My husband fully supports me in this decision.

I would like to assure you that I have sufficient funds to finance the trip and take care of the hospital expenses and doctors' fees.

I write to you in desperation and with a deep sense of urgency. Will you please accept my father as a patient on the terms outlined here? Please call me collect at your earliest convenience.

Sincerely yours,

Mary Park-Dent

Should Dr. Manuel accept Mrs. Park-Dent and her father as patients on the terms she proposes?

Case Discussion

(1) Background to Fetal Tissue Transplantation for Parkinson's Disease

(a) Parkinson's disease is a devastating neural disorder attributable to a degeneration of neurons in the region of the brain designated the substantia nigra. This degeneration inhibits the secretion of dopamine to regulate "normal" bodily movements. The characteristic features of Parkinson's disease include a mask-like facial expression, prominent trembling of the hands, arms or legs, stiffness of the extremities that limits movements, a rigid posture and a stiff gait. The cause of the disease is unknown and, at present, it is incurable.

(b) Experiments with fetal tissue transplants in mice, rats, and monkeys with artificially induced Parkinson's disease, reveal nerve regeneration that results in symptomatic relief. These boons are secured without significant adverse side effects in the experimental work done up to the present time. Because of the novelty of the procedure, the long range effects are not yet known.

The optimum time for fetal tissue transplantation is after the neurons have ceased to divide but prior to growing their long, fibrous axons.[1] Tissue implanted at this time is less likely to be rejected by the host's immune system.

(2) The Less Controversial Case of Fetal Tissue Transplantation

(a) Had Mrs. Park-Dent petitioned Dr. Manuel to treat her father with fetal tissue derived either from abortions for ectopic pregnancies or from elective abortions, her request would have been less problematic ethically for the team in Mexico than her proposal to terminate her child's life to alleviate her father's suffering. "Less problematic ethically" because of the existence of a context in which at least the crucial ethical issues had been addressed to the satisfaction of the appropriate committees at Hospital Salvador Mario. At this centre the great divide between animal and human research in the domain of fetal tissue transplantation had already been crossed. The procedure, approved by hospital ethics and research committees (subject to consent from patients and their relatives) had already been tried on human subjects with an acceptable degree of success in cell regeneration. The availability of fetal tissue from elective abortions testifies to the hospital's fairly liberal policy on abortion. Whether it would turn out to be liberal enough to honour Mrs. Park-Dent's request is moot. Whether it ought to be that liberal is one of the crucial moral worries of this case discussion.

(b) The main objections to fetal tissue transplantation come from those who hold a more conservative view of abortion. Certainly it makes a difference whether one views a fetus as a human being with potential rather than the equivalent of a bodily organ or a piece of cadaveric tissue. For those who hold a more elevated view of the fetus, the subsumption of fetal tissue transplantation under the anatomical tissue gift Acts adopted in North American jurisdictions is likely to be dismissed as inappropriate. Such Acts permit the donation of all or part of the human body at death. The dissimilarities between tissue and organ donation, on the one hand, and fetal tissue transplants, on the other, are claimed to outweigh the similarities, thus undermining the analogy alleged to hold between them. The putative dissimilarities are:

(i) As already noted, a fetus is not the equivalent of a kidney or a liver.

(ii) The term "donation" in this context is ambiguous. In straightforward cases of donation, the donors themselves donate their organs or bodily parts by means of advance directives. In the case of fetal tissue transplantation, however, the donation of fetal tissue is made by one individual on behalf of another. Hence the term "donor" is stretched beyond the boundaries of its customary usage. It is being made to do double duty for the decision-maker and the source of the donation.[2] In standard cases of donation, the decision-maker and the source of donation are identical. In fetal donation they are not.

(iii) But perhaps there is a better model than "direct consent"? What about surrogate consent involving minors? On this model a woman could then consent to tissue donation of a fetus she had elected to abort. Would that it were that clear-cut. Surrogate consent to treatment of minors is usually predicated on the continued existence of the children on whose behalf consent is given. By contrast, fetal tissue donation requires the demise or destruction of the fetus. This dissimilarity may be sufficient in itself to destroy the analogy between consenting to treatment of minors and consenting to fetal tissue donation.

(iv) Perhaps it would be more promising to compare giving permission for fetal tissue transplantation and giving permission for an autopsy on a minor. Whether or not the autopsy is performed on a minor is not essential to the point being made here. The qualifier "minor" is introduced simply to insure a closer similarity between the entities compared. The important point is that, in one crucial respect, the entities compared are on a par. What is done to either is not predicated on their continued existence. Both the child for autopsy and the fetus for tissue transplant are dead. Nevertheless, there is a crucial dissimilarity in the two cases. In authorizing an autopsy on an infant, the mother does not "elect" the death of the infant. Rather, the infant has died from other causes, usually natural ones. The same is not true of a woman who has elected to terminate her pregnancy and who is allowed a say in the disposal of the fetal remains. In such a case the woman who consents to the donation of fetal tissue has also requested the termination of her pregnancy.

One could try to get around this difficulty by insisting, as some ethicists do, that "the decision to abort disqualifies the mother from playing any role in the disposition of fetal remains."[3] The point being made is that "the ability of the 'proxy' to make an authentic gift of fetal tissue depends critically on the prior relation."[4] Where this disqualification leads depends on whether it is pursued by pro-life or pro-choice advocates. If advanced by a pro-life supporter it could lead to a ban on fetal tissue transplantation. If advocated by a pro-choice supporter it could lead to "routine salvage." Fetal tissue would be routinely harvested and used for promising medical interventions without seeking the woman's consent. Kathleen Nolan has misgivings about routine salvage. She insists that the moral acceptability of routine salvage of fetal materials should be made contingent on whether "routine salvage were standard for other cadavers."[5] But this is not the case. Our society has not endorsed routine salvage of organs or body tissue; nor is it clear on what ground it might endorse it unless on the ground that organs and body tissue belong to society rather than to individuals and their families. One envisages stiff resistance to such a proposal in a liberal democratic society like ours. The question to consider is whether such resistance is morally justifiable. In considering this question, consider the discussion surrounding the preceding case.

(3) The "Problematic" Case

Up to this point the difficulties in connection with fetal tissue transplantation have been confined to the so-called "less problematic" cases in which fetuses have already been slated for abortion. Proposals like that of Mrs. Park-Dent to abort a child for the purpose of treating someone else are likely to trigger deep concern. Even if, after deliberating over the troublesome questions raised in (2) above, we tend to favour the use of fetal tissue derived from elective abortions (whether routinely or with the woman's consent) on the grounds that abortion and the use of fetal tissue are distinct issues, that will not wash in the present case. For even if it could be argued in the case of elective abortions that "abortion and transplantation are practically and intentionally distinct rather than integrally related as means and ends,"[6] this distinction would not save the day for Mrs. Park-Dent. In her case the means-end link cannot be broken. Abortion is proposed in order to provide tissue for the relief of her father's suffering. Mrs. Park-Dent's proposal raises the question: "Does the relief of another's suffering constitute a proportionate reason for aborting a fetus?"

As the medical profession gears up for fetal-tissue transplantation some safeguards are beginning to emerge. These include: (i) no other source of viable tissue exists; (ii) the state of neurological impairment in the sufferer is a source of major tragedy for one proposing the abortion; (iii) the abortion decision is uncoerced; (iv) the male partner is supportive of the decision. Does the fact that Mrs. Park-Dent meets these criteria give her care-givers a green light to proceed? Before hastily offering an affirmative answer to that question, we should note that there is no mention whatsoever of the interests of the fetus in these proposed safeguards. Is that a serious omission? Recent challenges to the pro-choice position on the status of the fetus might lead us to suppose that it is. In these challenges to the pro-choice position on abortion, both in the United States and Canada, the stage of fetal development at which abortions are permissible is under discussion. There appears to be growing moral support for greater protection of the fetus later in the gestational process. If this support is translated into legislation it could have a profound effect on the issue of fetal tissue transplantation. The impact of revised abortion legislation on the fetal tissue transplantation issue is, of course, contingent on the "point" or "range" in gestational development at which therapeutic abortions would no longer be permissible. For effective transplantation, fetal tissue should be procured at the twelfth week. So if, for example, elective abortions were to be restricted to the first trimester, the need for twelve-week old fetuses (to insure effective transplantation) would locate abortion at the upper limit of the first trimester. The fact that the cut-off point for abortion on the first trimester criterion coincides with the optimum point for fetal tissue transplantation could lead to serious disagreement over Mrs. Park-Dent's proposal. The disagreement is not likely to be readily resolved by specifying a range rather than a point in the gestational process at which abortion becomes morally permissible. For even if one were to employ a range concept like "first trimester," as one reaches the upper limits of the range, the range tends to narrow to a point, in this case the twelfth week.

So, for fetal tissue transplantation to take place some flexibility with respect to the time limit on elective abortions is required. But this is an extremely controversial observation for it carries overtones of subordinating the point at which pregnancies may be terminated to the need to perform fetal tissue transplantation. Even many pro-choice advocates may experience difficulty with this ordering of priorities. Should the question about the "point" in the gestational process at which abortion should be allowed to take place not be settled independently of the need for tissue for transplantation? If not, won't the need for the fetal tissue prejudice the judgment in favour of subordinating any obligations we might have to protect the fetus to the needs of other sufferers? The unfinished moral agenda founders on whether we have obligations towards the fetus and, if so, at what point in the gestational process they arise.

In his book *Abortion and Moral Theory*, Wayne Sumner grounds obligations to the fetus in fetal sentience, which he argues allows "for the gradual emergence of moral standing in the order of nature."[7] As Sumner's thesis unfolds, however, it becomes clear that the emergence of moral standing does not occur early enough to present a challenge to the emerging practice of fetal transplantation. To do that it would need to be established that fetuses are sentient in the first trimester. Sentience would then serve to prohibit abortions at twelve weeks – the optimal point in the gestational process for tissue transplantation. Sumner, however, rules out sentience in the first trimester, assigns the fetus only a threshold status in the second trimester, and a minimal degree of sentience in the third trimester.[8] Whatever protections afforded the fetus on Sumner's view come too late in the gestational process to protect fetuses from abortions performed to provide tissue for transplantation. Does this give cause for alarm? Are there still some lingering doubts about the moral propriety of aborting fetuses in order to provide tissue for transplantation? If so, are these doubts attributable to cultural lag, to a failure of nerve, or to what?

In discussing the pros and cons of fetal tissue procurement Dr. Alan Fine favours prohibiting the donation of fetal tissue to any specific recipient.[9] This proposed prohibition has an immediate bearing on Mrs. Park-Dent's proposal to donate fetal tissue to her father. Actually, there are two issues that converge here. If tissue donation is restricted to elective abortions, then – because they use donors who are not blood-related to the recipient – problems of tissue in-compatibility and rejection are more likely to arise. The possibility of this happening could account for the peculiar nature of the request made by a woman in a story carried by the *New York Times*. She asked to be inseminated with her father's sperm to provide him with compatible fetal tissue for a therapeutic neural transplant.[10] And what about the prospect of women selling their fetuses for commercial profit? If we allow women to sell fetuses for therapeutic purposes, should we also allow them to sell their fetuses for purposes of medical research? Is there no end to the ramifications of fetal tissue transplantation once one steps onto the slippery slope? Can we establish a footing on this slippery slope to prevent further slide, or should we refrain from stepping on it in the first place?

In considering these questions, ask yourself whether you agree with the following conclusions of Canada's Royal Commission on New Reproductive and Genetic Technologies. The conclusions deal with the use of fetal tissue for research purposes. But at least some of them might apply to situations where the purposes are largely therapeutic.

On the basis of the evidence reviewed by the Commission, there is a real possibility that research involving the use of fetal tissue could result in considerable alleviation of human suffering. At present, elective abortion provides the only practical source of fetal tissue. Research carried out under the controlled conditions we have specified may benefit human health and is respectful of human dignity.

The controlled conditions for obtaining and using fetal tissue include safeguards against coercion, commercialization, and unethical use of fetal tissue. We recommend: prohibition of giving or receiving payment for fetal tissue; consent to use of tissue obtained separately from and subsequent to the decision to have an abortion; standards of information disclosure; and the method of abortion to be chosen for the woman's safety and health only. We recommend licensing by [a National Reproductive Technologies Commission] of any provider of fetal tissue, with conditions of license to ensure that fetal tissue is obtained in accordance with the above licensing requirements and is only provided for use in research directed to understanding biologic mechanisms with potential relevance to treating disease.[11]

Notes

1   Alan Fine, "The Ethics of Fetal Tissue Transplants," *Hastings Centre Report*, 5 (1988), 5.
2   Kathleen Nolan, "*Genug ist Genug*: A Fetus Is Not a Kidney," *Hastings Centre Report*, 6 (1988), 19.
3   John A. Robertson, "Rights Symbolism, and Public Policy in Fetal Tissue Transplants," in *Hastings*, 9.
4   Nolan, 14.
5   Nolan, 15.
6   Mary B. Mahowald et.al., "Ethical Options in Fetal Transplants," *Hastings Centre Report*, 1 (1987), 13.
7   L.W. Sumner, *Abortion and Moral Theory* (New Jersey: Princeton University Press, 1981), 144.
8   Sumner, 149.
9   Fine, 7.
10 Fine, 6.
11 Royal Commission on New Reproductive Technologies, *Final Report: Summary and Highlights*, (Ottawa: Canada Communication Group Publishing, 1993.)

Chapter 11: AIDS

Case 11:1 Fear of Contracting AIDS at a Community College

Susan Smith is a faculty member at Spencer Community College. Susan began as an instructor in the School's Department of Early Childhood Education and worked her way up to Department Chairperson. Following a stellar performance in the latter role, Susan was promoted to Academic Vice-President of the College. Six months into her appointment, Susan was summoned to the office of the College President, who had an unusual task for her. She was to prepare a discussion paper on AIDS at Spencer College. A certain number of faculty and staff had expressed serious concern that the College was not doing enough to protect its members from HIV (Human Immunodeficiency Virus), the virus which causes AIDS (Acquired Immunodeficiency Syndrome). There was also concern that the College might unwittingly be sending HIV-infected students out into the community. Spencer College has an innovative co-op system of instruction in Early Childhood Education. This system allows students to spend one-third of their school year in preschool settings gaining valuable hands-on experience. The President wanted Susan to prepare a report which addressed the concerns expressed. More specifically, she was to address the following questions. Should there be mandatory HIV testing at the College for all actual and potential faculty, staff, and students? Should HIV-infected individuals be barred from the College? If not, should the identity of people known to have AIDS or to be infected with HIV be revealed to the College community?

Susan was faced with a daunting task. The result was the following report, which was to serve as a basis for discussion before the College's Board of Governors.

Case Discussion

Report: AIDS at Spencer College

By: Susan Smith, Academic Vice-President

This report is divided into three parts. In Section A, I outline certain key facts about AIDS and how it is contracted. The intention is to ensure that the College's response to AIDS is as informed and intelligent as possible. It is an unfortunate fact that many moral arguments relating to AIDS pay far too little attention to the relevant facts. As a consequence there is considerable muddled thinking and irrational behaviour – a tragic consequence when so much is at stake. In Section B, I will outline briefly the basic value conflicts which lie at the heart of debates about AIDS and AIDS policy. Analogies will be drawn which suggest that reactions to AIDS are often over-reactions precipitated by ignorance, irrational fears, and fallacious thinking. Finally, in Section C, I will address the specific questions raised by the President.

Section A: AIDS and HIV

"AIDS" stands for Acquired Immunodeficiency Syndrome. AIDS is caused by a virus called HIV (Human Immunodeficiency Virus) which attacks and seriously disrupts the body's immune system, its defence against disease. If HIV gets into a person's blood it infects, and may destroy, certain white blood cells called helper-T cells. These white blood cells enable the body to ward off disease. Without the protection of their immune system, people with AIDS suffer from fatal infections and cancers.

The term "AIDS" describes only the most serious form of HIV infection. HIV infection is a progressive disease, with the seriousness of the symptoms and complications increasing as the immune system becomes weaker with the passage of time. When HIV infection begins, there may be no obvious symptoms and the infected person may appear healthy for many years. Researchers believe that a number of as yet unknown factors, in addition to HIV, may be necessary to trigger "full-blown AIDS."

The time-line for the development of full-blown AIDS is as follows:[1]

1. Exposure: 2-6 weeks after infection, individuals experience Acute

HIV Syndrome. In this period, the individual has fevers, headaches, sore throat, and rashes. No specific indicator diseases are present. During the first six months following exposure, antibodies for the HIV virus cannot usually be found in the body. T-cell counts are normal.

2. Asymptomatic period: This may last several years. No symptoms of the illness are present. The infected person feels healthy and may be unaware of the infection. At this time, the virus is replicating in the T-cells and the T-cell count steadily declines. Antibodies for HIV are now detectable.

3. Symptomatic period: This may also last several years. Individuals begin to contract symptoms for "indicator diseases," HIV count increases dramatically, and T-cell count is low.

4. Onset of AIDS: At this state, the patient is positively diagnosed with one or more of AIDS indicator diseases and T-cell counts have dropped to a very low level.

5. Death: T-cell count is close to zero, and the person's immune response to diseases and tumours is very poor.

The time from the diagnosis of AIDS to the time of death varies widely. The average life-span after AIDS diagnosis is roughly two years.[2]

AIDS symptoms are not specific to the disease but are like those of many other medical conditions. General symptoms include: swollen lymph glands in the neck, armpit or groin; night sweats or fevers; loss of weight for no apparent reason; severe tiredness; thrush, a thick persistent whitish coating on the tongue or throat; and diarrhoea. In most cases, these general symptoms are caused by common illnesses and not by HIV infection itself, but the latter renders the body particularly susceptible to them. As noted, the most severe stage of HIV infection is AIDS, which may develop only after many years. At this extreme stage of the infection, the immune system has been so severely damaged that many life-threatening, indicator diseases appear. Some of the most common diseases developed by people with AIDS include Kaposi's sarcoma, a rare skin cancer; Pneumocystis carinii pneumonia (PCP), an unusual lung infection that causes a persistent shortness of breath and a heavy persistent cough; Hodgkin's disease, cancer of the lymph organs; and brain infection, direct damage to the brain cells caused by HIV infection and resulting in loss of concentration, confusion, and disorientation.

Anyone who sets out to research the relevant literature on AIDS and HIV will be astonished by the unanimity among informed sources concerning the means by which HIV can be contracted. Such unanimity is rare within scientific circles. Virtually all sources are in agreement that the disease is communicable only by intimate sexual contact, by shared contaminated needles, by the injection of infected blood or blood products, and across the placenta from mother to infant. (According to current estimates, an HIV infected mother has a 25-35 per cent chance of passing the virus to her unborn child.) Casual contact with an infected person, whether symptomatic or asymptomatic, has not been found to transmit HIV. This includes hand shaking; sharing common drinking glasses, clothing, or toilets; and sharing "airspace." Transmission of HIV appears to require direct inoculation of the virus into the bloodstream. In fact, there is good evidence that even prolonged and close familial exposure to persons infected with HIV will not result in transmission of the virus.

It is generally agreed that one cannot catch AIDS from "casual contact." With the exception of sexual partners, people in households with AIDS patients do not get the virus. Medical personnel caring for AIDS patients get AIDS only under highly unusual circumstances, as when a British nurse accidentally injected herself some years ago with infected blood. (Her AIDS was not conclusively linked to the needle-stick injury.) Medical personnel who are bitten by AIDS patients suffering from dementia do not become infected. No child has been shown to transmit the infection to another child at school or at home. There is general agreement that the virus is not transmitted by bed-bugs, mosquitos, saliva, urine (changing diapers), toilet seats, sharing cups, breathing, hugging, or other household means.

It is clear that aside from cases involving sex, direct blood injection, and birth (HIV being transmitted from mother to fetus across the placenta), circumstances have to be quite extraordinary before HIV can be transmitted. AIDS is indeed a "communicable disease" but it is not even close to being a highly "infectious" or "contagious" disease on a par with typhoid, smallpox, or yellow fever. Despite this, AIDS is too often thought of as highly infectious, as a disease which can be transmitted through simple touching or by sharing air-space with infected persons. It's as if the virus's potentially lethal consequences blind people to the fact that it is virtually impossible to contract HIV except in very special ways. The HIV virus cannot be transmitted by casual contact of the sort one might experience at home, in a store, in a cafeteria, or in a college classroom. Within these settings non-infected persons are in fact far more a risk to people with HIV than the other way round. Catching a truly infectious virus such as the flu can be fatal for a person with AIDS.

An important point about AIDS worth stressing is that only some people with HIV infection also have AIDS. HIV takes time to develop to its final stage: AIDS. The result is that people who test positive for HIV antibodies are not necessarily going to die right away. Many seem to go on to lead fairly normal lives for a considerable period of time. This is true, for example, of the famous basketball player, Magic Johnston, who continues to lead a relatively normal life in the absence of (serious) symptoms.

Yet another crucial fact about AIDS is that it has catastrophic social implications for its victims. People infected with HIV, particularly those who have developed AIDS, are often subject to loss of livelihood, ostracism from the community, denial of insurance, eviction notices from landlords, refusals by morticians to prepare bodies for burial, and exclusions of children from schools. These consequences result not merely from unwarranted fear, but from homophobia and other kinds of moral prejudice. One sometimes hears the comment that AIDS is the natural, indeed divinely ordained, consequence of unnatural activities like drug abuse and homosexuality. Homosexuals, prostitutes and intravenous drug users evoke widespread moral condemnation of their lifestyles by others. The result is often discrimination, social isolation, cruelty, and flagrant denials of the freedom and autonomy cherished by human beings.

Section B: The Basic Value Conflicts

At bottom, ethical questions surrounding our responses to HIV involve an age old conflict between two sets of competing moral considerations. On the one hand there is the need to respect individual rights to such things as liberty, autonomy, privacy, and (perhaps) sufficient opportunities to engage in meaningful activities. For want of a better word, we can refer to this somewhat heterogeneous collection of rights as "autonomy rights." On the other hand, there is a no less important right, sometimes said to reside in the public at large, to be free from the harmful effects of individuals and their activities. We can refer to this negative, passive right by the phrase "security right." It is important to be aware that the conflict between autonomy and security rights is a familiar one. It is at the centre of such issues as the conditions under which people should be allowed to pursue hazardous activities like fireworks displays, automobile racing and owning pit-bull terriers. It also lies at the heart of other, less glamorous but no less important questions such as where speed limits and blood/alcohol levels (for drivers) should be set. It is unquestionable that the number of fatal or debilitating car accidents would decrease were the speed limit on four-lane, divided highways halved. Despite this we have chosen to opt for the much higher speed limits now in force, with full knowledge that we are thereby threatening the security rights of many innocent people. Many more people die than would do so were the speed limits lower. We accept this, however, presumably out of respect for individual autonomy rights and other things of social value, such as quick transportation of perishable goods.

The example of speed limits is an instructive one. It illustrates not only the extent to which security rights compete with autonomy rights within our societies, but also the important fact that *security rights do not always trump autonomy rights*. It is quite often the other way round. Much depends in such cases on judgments concerning the value of the activities protected by autonomy rights and the degree of risk those activities create for other people. In both morality and law, such judgments are often expressed in terms of the "reasonableness" or "unreasonableness" of the risks incurred. If the risks are thought to be reasonable, the autonomy rights will be held to outweigh the security rights; unreasonable, and it will be the other way round. Sometimes, of course, a compromise is reached. People are allowed to pursue their desire to race fast cars, but only under conditions which minimize the acknowledged risk of harm to innocent bystanders. People are also allowed to drive at high speeds on highways, under conditions which allow for even greater risk of harm to innocent bystanders. This is no doubt because racing cars is a less valuable activity than reaching one's destination in a "reasonable" amount of time. The greater value attached to the latter activity leads us to accept the much greater risk. Many more people are killed on highways than on the sidelines of race-tracks, but we're willing to live with this fact for the sake of the competing values.

The implications of the foregoing analysis for the questions concerning social responses to HIV infection should be fairly clear. Speaking quite generally, HIV infection represents a standard conflict between the victim's autonomy rights and the security rights of those who might be infected through contact with her. And so the question to be addressed is not simply whether HIV victims are a threat to innocent people, but whether the risks they create are reasonable or unreasonable. As with any conflict between security and autonomy, it is not enough simply to point out that individuals with HIV pose a risk to innocent people. As suggested earlier, our society accepts such risks all the time – if they are reasonable ones. And whether a risk is reasonable or not is a function of its degree and the value of what is threatened if autonomy rights are abrogated or enforced.

Once the issues are seen in this light, answers to moral questions posed by HIV in an educational setting like a college or pre-school begin to emerge. The risk of contracting HIV through casual contact of the sort experienced in such educational settings is extremely minimal. To be sure, the consequences of actually catching the virus in that, or any other, setting can be catastrophic. Not only will the victim be in danger of developing AIDS; he or she will also be subject to the wide variety of undesirable social consequences noted earlier.

The gravity of these potential consequences no doubt weighs heavily in people's thinking – and so it should. But it is a universally accepted principle of rationality that the seriousness of a possible consequence must be discounted by the degree of probability that it will actually occur, which in this case is virtually nil. The probability of contracting AIDS in a normal educational setting, including a preschool setting, is so slight that the actual, as opposed to the imagined, risks to innocent bystanders are all but non-existent. When we conjoin this fact with the virtual certainty that seriously harmful consequences will result from things like screening all faculty, staff, and students for HIV, revealing the names of HIV carriers to fellow students, or refusing admission to applicants who test positive, answers become clear. The autonomy rights (and indeed, in some cases involving extreme prejudice, the security rights) of HIV victims must, within the contexts in question, take precedence. Factors such as paranoia and moral prejudice should not be allowed to cloud our moral judgments. At a time in the lives of AIDS sufferers when they are most in need of our compassion, concern, and support, it would be a cruel dereliction of moral duty were we to allow ignorance, irrational fears, and prejudice to influence our judgments. This point is of even greater relevance in the present case. As an institute of higher learning, Spencer College has an especially weighty responsibility not to base its policies and decisions on ignorance and prejudice.

Section C: Five Questions

I would like briefly to address the specific policy issues raised by the College President. I will do so by posing and answering five key questions.

1. Should there be a compulsory HIV testing procedure in place for all applicants to and students of Spencer College?

The answer is clearly no. Excepting sex, direct inoculation, and childbirth, circumstances must be quite extraordinary before transmission of HIV can occur. What purpose would such an extremely costly testing procedure serve? Within a classroom, or any other setting typical of a Community College, the chances of HIV transmission are so negligible as to be almost non-existent. Since there are no unreasonable risks involved, there is no need to know whether a person has HIV infection. So why should Spencer College try to gather such information? The testing procedure would be costly, serve no useful purpose, violate the privacy of HIV victims, and increase the chance of undesirable social consequences for the HIV carrier.

There is also the problem of "false positive." Techniques for detecting the presence of HIV have become very sophisticated. The risk that an individual's HIV test will falsely come up positive is extremely small. Nevertheless, the possibility must still be acknowledged. Given the traumatic consequences for a person falsely labelled an HIV carrier, one requires a very good reason indeed to require testing. There is no such reason.

2. If no such general procedure is warranted, should compulsory testing be in place for applicants to the Department of Early Childhood Education?

Again, there is no need. As with a college setting, there is virtually no risk within a preschool setting that a teacher will accidentally infect a student. There is therefore no valid reason at all for the College to know whether one of its student-teachers has HIV. Of course it's always possible for such a student teacher to infect a child knowingly and intentionally. But it is also possible for such a person intentionally to harm students in all sorts of other ways.

3. Whether or not the College should itself require HIV testing of any of its members, should it nevertheless refuse admission or continued membership to individuals who are known to have the HIV virus?

Absolutely not. As before, we need to stress that such individuals pose no threat to others within a normal College setting. There is no just basis, then, for denying them the educational opportunities they seek. It is perhaps important here to note the difference between a person with AIDS and a person infected with HIV. The latter may earn a College degree and engage in meaningful and productive employment for years before developing AIDS. Given that individuals infected with HIV pose no unreasonable risk to other members of the College, it would not only be a violation of their autonomy rights, but a waste of a valuable human resource to deny them membership in the College. As for those with AIDS, they may yet have occasion for rewarding and productive activity. It would be cruelty of the highest degree to deny such individuals opportunities which give meaning to what little life they have left.

4. If individuals with HIV or AIDS should not be denied membership in the College, should they nevertheless be required to inform other members of the College of their condition – or must the infected member's right of confidentiality take precedence?

In response, one might reasonably ask: What possible purpose could be served by a requirement of disclosure? And if a purpose is served, is it sufficiently important to require individuals infected with HIV to shoulder the awesome burden of discrimination, denials of autonomy rights – and sometimes even security rights? Once we are clear about how HIV can be transmitted, the costs of mandatory disclosure will be seen to far outweigh any possible advantages. Confidentiality is a cherished commodity in social life. It is crucial within the areas of medicine and disease, particularly when the disease in question is one which attracts the kind of irrationality and prejudice associated with AIDS and HIV.

This is not to say, of course, that an individual infected with HIV is never under obligation to disclose his or her illness to another person. This would certainly be true if the two intended to become sexual partners or to share an intravenous needle. It is the responsibility of the individuals involved, however, to ensure that this information is communicated between them. One would hope that Spencer College considers the private sexual affairs of its staff and students well beyond the scope of its concern.

5. Should HIV testing be part of the recruitment process for faculty and staff at Spencer College?

Why? Again, the threat posed is negligible. Should the College be testing possible recruits for emotional instability, sexual deviance, or violent tendencies because people who fall within these categories might harm someone? Should the College exclude former hockey players because hockey is sometimes a violent game which may attract individuals with violent tendencies? If not, then why should the College single out those who test positive for HIV?

"True," someone might say. "But what about the pension and group insurance plans, and long-range planning regarding the number of faculty and staff needed to mount the various College programs? We do not want to hire people only to see them die shortly thereafter. Should we not be concerned with the economic and strategic consequences of allowing HIV carriers to join the ranks?"

Yes we should, but not to the point of excluding them from employment. Consider the following points. First, people with HIV infection often lead reasonably long and productive lives. A person with HIV isn't necessarily going to die tomorrow or even next year. HIV is not the same as AIDS. Secondly, if we deny employment to people with HIV, should we do the same for people with high blood pressure, heart disease or bad eating habits? Should we be tracing family histories to see if there is any evidence of alcohol abuse in the families of applicants? After all, a person who comes from an environment in which alcohol is abused is more likely than one who does not to be an unsatisfactory and unreliable employee. He is also more likely to be a drain on the medical plan. Should we therefore be probing the family histories of individuals and turning down high-risk people because they're bad risks for the pension and medical plans? If the answer is no, then why are things different when it comes to HIV infection? Employing individuals infected with HIV does not clearly pose a significantly greater risk to the group plans and long-range College strategies than employing people with high blood pressure and family histories of heart disease or alcohol abuse. The exclusion of all HIV carriers would be highly discriminatory and wasteful of valuable human resources.

"True," it might be said, "but what about people who not only have HIV but AIDS as well? They will in all likelihood be unable to fulfil their duties. But if they are unable to fulfil their duties then we should not be hiring them."

That someone is unable to fulfil her duties is a good reason for denying her employment. But not all people with AIDS are unable to fulfil their employment duties. Those who are able to work should not be denied the opportunity to do so. Such a denial would be discriminatory. Those who are truly unable to meet the legitimate requirements of the job should not be allowed to try if the interests of others (say the students who will not be receiving adequate instruction) are being seriously compromised. But then the grounds for relieving the person of her job lies not in the fact that she has AIDS, but in the fact that she is unable to perform the required tasks. There is nothing discriminatory here – and nothing to suggest a policy of not hiring people just because they have AIDS.

Further Reflections and Questions

Do you agree with Susan Smith's answers to the key questions regarding this case? Are the issues really as clear cut as her argument seems to suppose? Suppose that the issues did not concern college membership but rather the right of a surgeon to continue operating on patients once she had been diagnosed with HIV? In this instance there is a possibility that the surgeon might nick herself and spill infected blood into the patient's open wound. Double-gloving can help, but it cannot eliminate the risk altogether. Are the risks here too high to allow the surgeon to operate? If not, must the patient be made fully aware of the risks involved?

Notes

1   The following information is derived from an unpublished report by Ayumi Goto, "HIV Education: Learning and Living with AIDS in the Upper West Region, Ghana." Goto's source is Abbas, Andrew and Jordan, *Cellular and Molecular Immunology*, 2nd ed. (Philadelphia: W.B. Saunders Co., 1996). I hereby express my thanks to Ms. Goto.

2   Goto, 14.

Case 11:2 Canada's Tainted Blood Scandal

(1) Report on a Tragedy

On November 26, 1997, Mr. Justice Horace Krever released his long-awaited Report of the Commission of Inquiry on the Blood System in Canada (the Krever Report). The Report had been commissioned by the Federal Government of Canada in response to public outcry over the perceived negligence of government and Red Cross officials in dealing with mounting evidence that HIV and Hepatitis C were being spread through the blood supply system. The Krever Report, four years in the making, included three volumes, was 1200 pages in length, and was based on over 50,000 pages of testimony from 427 witnesses.

In his Report, Justice Krever does not assign blame to any specific individuals for their role in the tainted blood tragedy, nor does he recommend that individuals who contracted AIDS or Hepatitis C through tainted blood be compensated financially. Krever does, however, chronicle a large-scale "systemic failure" which led to an estimated 1,200 Canadians being infected with HIV. This number includes only those who received the virus directly through blood or blood products, but does not include friends or family members who were subsequently infected through sexual contact, maternal transmission, or other means. Twelve thousand is the generally accepted figure for individuals directly infected through the blood supply with Hepatitis C. Krever estimates, however, that the true number may exceed 60,000.

(2) Highlights

Among the highlights of the Krever Report are the following claims:[1]

(i)   The federal government of Canada did not properly monitor the activities of the Canadian Red Cross.
(ii) The federal government reacted far too slowly and cautiously to the threat of blood-born HIV, mistakenly and negligently downplaying the risks to Canadians of becoming infected by tainted blood.[2]
(iii) The provincial governments, which funded the Red Cross blood programme, failed to provide adequate funding for scientific

tests which could have screened out blood tainted with HIV and Hepatitis C.

(iv) The provincial governments failed to take adequate measures to track down infected individuals, some of whom were unaware of their infection and unknowingly passed the virus on to their sexual partners or children. Government bureaucrats "appear to have been more concerned about preventing public questioning about the safety of the blood system and deflecting controversy" than with providing adequate information.

(v) The Red Cross failed to take sufficient steps to institute a programme to screen out high-risk donors, e.g., sexually active gay men.

(vi) The Red Cross failed to replace its supply of contaminated blood product with newer, heat-treated products which were free of contamination. Instead they waited till the contaminated supply was exhausted before introducing the safer products.

(vii) The Red Cross took far too long to prepare a pamphlet about the nature and transmission of HIV and AIDS. According to Krever, the actions of the Red Cross were "slow and bureaucratic."

(viii) The pamphlet that the Red Cross did finally produce was vague and confusing.

(ix) Of the 28,000 estimated cases of Hepatitis C that occurred after 1986, when a reliable test of its presence was adopted in the United States but rejected in Canada for reasons of cost/efficiency, 85 per cent could have been avoided.

(3) Recommendations

Among the 50 recommendations made in the Krever Report are the following:

(i) The Canadian blood supply system should be governed by five principles:
  1. Blood should be treated as a public resource.
  2. Blood donors should not be paid.
  3. Canada should be self-sufficient in its blood supply.
  4. There should be free, universal access to blood.
  5. Safety should be paramount.
(ii) A single, independent blood authority should be created.

At the time of this writing, a new agency called the "Canadian Blood System" has been created with $81 million supplied by the federal government. The operations of the CBS are to be funded by the provinces and the territories, and it will have full control over Canada's blood supply. Its activities will include soliciting blood donations, overseeing appropriate screening processes, and educating the public on issues of health and safety.

Case Discussion

(1) A Basis for Reflection

As noted above, the Krever Report is some 1200 pages in length and includes a multitude of complex details chronicling a perceived failure expeditiously to halt the spread of HIV and Hepatitis C through the Canadian blood supply. The Report is essentially one (highly respected) individual's informed assessment of a multi-faceted situation in which many individuals and many systemic factors contributed to a tragedy. Judgments of fault and blame, both moral and legal, are in such instances highly contestable, and "facts" are very much subject to interpretation. Although Justice Krever fought for, and was granted by the Supreme Court of Canada, the right to "name names" in his report, he did not assign blame to specific individuals, angering some advocacy groups who viewed this as a lost opportunity. At the time of this writing, the Royal Canadian Mounted Police are still considering whether to lay criminal charges against certain individuals whose decisions were at the centre of the blood scandal.

In view of all these factors, it would be irresponsible to include a detailed analysis of the tainted blood scandal. Instead, we provide below a short excerpt from the Krever Report which can serve as a basis for reflection and discussion. In reading through the extract, try to imagine yourself in the position of a Red Cross official, with a large bank of blood and blood products for which there is always urgent need but which you know might be, to some unknown degree, infected with HIV and Hepatitis C. You have seen what other countries have done, but you believe that decisions should be taken not because they mimic what others have decided, but because they are correct. Try to imagine how you would weigh the relevant factors in coming to a decision. In so doing, you might consider it useful to consider some of the points made above in Cases 9:1 and 9:2, which deal with dialysis machine shortages and budget-cutting in neonatology. Bear in mind as well the various points made in the preceding case, 11:1, especially those concerning the evaluation of risks and the basic value conflicts which underlie any such exercise. Finally, give whatever weight you think appropriate to the following brief observations.

When doing or evaluating "pure" science, in an environment in which pressures to find immediate answers are absent, we have the luxury of waiting for practical certainty. Often conclusions will be rejected in science unless their probability is greater than 95 per cent as calculated using some generally agreed mathematical procedure. This means that conclusions in which many individuals have the utmost confidence will not be accepted by scientists because the requisite degree of "proof" has yet to be achieved. When time is not of the essence, this extreme caution in accepting hypotheses is fully warranted.

Consider, now, the hypotheses which were relevant in the present case. They concerned, for example, the nature and cause of AIDS and Hepatitis C; the means through which these diseases can be spread; the degree to which they were present in existing supplies of blood and blood products; and the chances of someone being infected by tainted blood or blood products were they supplied from existing sources. Would it have been right not to act on any of these hypotheses until such time as the usual level of scientific proof had been achieved? Presumably not. But then what is the appropriate level of confidence? In answering this last question, which involves one essentially in what is often called "risk analysis," it would be appropriate to consider the time and resources required to create new supplies of blood and blood products in which these diseases are absent; what would be involved in providing alternative services to those for whom immediate supplies of blood or blood products were necessary; what might otherwise be done with the resources needed to deal with a situation in which all current sources of blood and blood products are destroyed; the social consequences of loss of faith in the blood supply system (which Justice Krever thought was a factor leading the relevant governments to delay tracking high-risk recipients); and finally, but perhaps most importantly, the devastating impact upon infected individuals (and their friends and families) who would otherwise not have received infected blood were the old supply destroyed, more vigorous screening to take place, and a much greater effort put into public education.

In developing your thoughts on these matters, keep in mind one final point: hindsight is 20/20. That a decision turned out, in retrospect, to be one which caused great harm does not necessarily mean that the agent did the wrong thing, or that she is to be blamed for her conduct. On some deontological theories, it is the agent's intentions which matter, not the consequences of her actions. But even if consequences do matter, we must still bear in mind that the full facts of a situation are often unknown. We do not always know the consequences which either will, or are likely to, follow from our decisions. In other words, when determining what we ought to do we cannot occupy the God's-eye view. Rather we must work in partial ignorance and base our decisions on the evidence available to us. As a result, it is possible, in the absence of full knowledge, to cause great harm by doing what, at the time, *appeared to be* the right thing to do, *appeared to be* the course of action which would bring about the best consequences. In judging individuals, one must always bear in mind what it was that they knew at the time they acted, and what it was that they ought to have known when they chose their course of action. We can look back now, at the mid 1980s, and see that it would clearly have been better had the Canadian officials done what the Americans had done. But whether, given what they knew or ought to have known at the time, they can be blamed for their conduct is perhaps an open question.

(2) Excerpt from The Final Report of the Commission of Inquiry on the Blood System in Canada[3]

In late 1982 and early 1983, after more than a year of exponential growth in the AIDS epidemic, evidence indicated that the causative agent of AIDS was present in the U.S. blood supply. By this time, AIDS was also occurring in Canada, but no cases had, as yet, been attributed to the Canadian blood supply. The rate of reported AIDS in Canada was the highest of any country except the United States and Haiti. Senior scientists in Canada estimated that the progress of the epidemic in Canada was 1 1/2 years behind that in the United States. Canadians thus had a vital opportunity to take preventative measures against the transmission of AIDS, including transmission through blood transfusion.

Although other institutions were involved in the blood system, the Red Cross had the primary responsibility for implementing measures to reduce the risk of transfusion-associated AIDS in Canada, just as it had developed measures for other diseases transmissible by blood. Unfortunately, the measures taken by the Red Cross in response to the risk of transfusion-associated AIDS between 1983 and the summer of 1985 were ineffective and half-hearted. Its actions were characterized by a refusal to accept and act upon risks to which prudent blood services, elsewhere in the world, were responding. Canada thus lost the opportunity given by the 1 1/2 years by which the epidemic in this country trailed that in the United States.

In Canada, the federal government regulated the manufacture of blood products and the collection of plasma by plasmapheresis, but it did not actively regulate the collection and processing of whole blood. Unlike its U.S. counterpart, the Department of National Health and Welfare never issued guidelines or recommendations for the collection of blood in Canada. Until the summer of 1985, neither the federal government nor the provincial governments gave the Red Cross directions or showed any leadership in helping the Red Cross to cope with issues of transfusion-associated AIDS.

It can fairly be said that the national office of the Canadian Red Cross was as well informed about the U.S. blood system as were most U.S. blood bankers. Although the Canadian Red Cross did not have the benefit of assistance and direction from governments in Canada with respect to measures to reduce the risk of transfusion-associated AIDS, it was aware of the guidelines and recommendations issued by the U.S. governmental authorities for blood banks in that country.

Because of these similarities and because of the fact that Canada possessed one of the highest reported rates of AIDS in the world, one would have expected the Canadian Red Cross to follow the measures for risk reduction that had been adopted in the United States or to develop equally effective measures of its own for reducing the risk.

There is no reasonable explanation for the length of time it took the Canadian Red Cross to prepare the pamphlet about AIDS, particulary when it is compared to the time it took other blood services throughout the world to prepare pamphlets or information sheets for donors. Blood collectors in the United States put pamphlets in place within days of being told to do so by the Department of Health and Human Services. European countries that had not already done so followed suit in the spring and early summer of 1983, soon after similar recommendations were made by the Council of Europe.

The [Canadian] Red Cross development of a pamphlet was slow

and bureaucratic.

The pamphlet that was finally distributed in the spring of 1984 for use at blood donation clinics, moreover, contained an outmoded description of persons at high risk of contracting AIDS. It referred to "homosexual or bisexual men with multiple partners." This language was vague and confusing.

Dr. Perraults's message to the board and medical directors also repeated the statement that there were no "officially recognized cases of transfusion-associated AIDS cases in Canada." Unofficial transfusion-associated AIDS cases were beginning to surface.

When AIDS first appeared, public health officials understood that there had never been a sexually transmitted disease known to be transmitted homosexually that was not also transmitted heterosexually.

The managers of the blood transfusion service were rightly concerned, and in consequence developed two views about inventory management that affected the conversion to heat-treated concentrates.

Its officials accordingly developed an implementation plan that included the exhaustion of the inventory.

It is clear that the Red Cross managers interpreted the assurance to mean that the Red Cross would be allowed to continue distributing the non-heat-treated concentrates until they were exhausted, for they created an implementation plan that included exhaustion of the non-heat-treated concentrates that were in inventory and in process even if heat-treated concentrates were obtained before the old stock was exhausted.

The exhaustion of the non-heat-treated inventory was linked to the accumulation of a reserve of heat-treated concentrates; the longer the introduction of the new concentrates was delayed in order to exhaust the old inventory, the greater would be the stock of the new concentrates when the transitional period ended.

On 21 November 1984, long before the May-June 1985 transitional period began, the Red Cross told Cutter (Laboratories) not to deliver heat-treated factor VIII concentrate or, if it did deliver them, that the labelling of the concentrates should not reveal that they were heat treated. The instruction was given the day after Dr. Derek Naylor wrote his memorandum linking the timing of the conversions to the exhaustion of the non-heat-treated concentrates.

Notes

1 Some of these are summarized in an article by Mark Kennedy, published in *The Ottawa Citizen*, November 26, 1997.

2 The following are some relevant dates as reported by the Canadian Press on August 2, 1997.

July, 1981: AIDS is first identified among homosexuals in California;

July, 1982: AIDS is first identified in hemophiliacs;

December, 1982: AIDS is identified in blood transfusion recipients;

May, 1983: HIV is isolated as the virus which causes AIDS;

June 1983: Blood transfusions are recognized as a "risk" factor for AIDS;

November, 1985: The Canadian Red Cross starts screening all blood for HIV;

During 1987: Guidelines adopted in the United States and Canada to encourage individuals who had transfusions to be tested for HIV;

February, 1994: Krever Inquiry begins.

3 Published by Public Works and Government Services Canada, November, 1997.

Chapter 12: Unanalyzed Cases for Further Study

Case 12:1 Should Cattle Prods Be Used to Correct Self-Destructive Behaviour?

Jeremy was a 21-year-old profoundly retarded man with powerful self-destructive compulsions. He was speechless and partially blind. In the past Jeremy had bitten chunks of flesh out of his knees and arms; his back, chest, and ribs were covered in bruises. He would pull his hair, bite his wrists, bang his forehead against walls and tables, and slap himself repeatedly in the face. He would sometimes deliver ferocious blows with his fists to the area between his eyes. One result of Jeremy's compulsive behaviour was a badly deformed ear. The precise cause of the self-injurious conduct was unknown, though some of the specialists at the Northwest Regional Centre for the Mentally Retarded suspected it had to do with Jeremy's desire for attention.

Unrestrained, Jeremy was completely unmanageable. When he first came to the Northwest Centre, his self-destructive compulsions were so strong that he would probably have managed to kill himself had he been left alone for a hour. According to the Director of the Centre, "He could do so much damage so fast that we had to have two staff with him at all times." In the initial stages of Jeremy's treatment at the Centre, various techniques were used and proved partially successful. For instance, early on Jeremy was made to sit at a table with his left arm restrained and his right arm in the grasp of a staff member. A row of Smarties was placed before him. The staff member would allow Jeremy's arm to move towards the Smarties, which he was allowed to eat. But the moment he tried to strike himself, the arm would be grabbed tightly while another staff member sprayed cold water onto Jeremy's face. This technique worked for a time, but after a few weeks its effectiveness ceased. Other techniques, involving both positive and negative reinforcement, were employed by the Centre, but none seemed to offer any hope of correcting Jeremy's destructive compulsions.

After considerable soul-searching, the staff decided to try more aversive therapy. The device used was a modified electric cattle prod with a force of 150 volts. The prod produces a very unpleasant sensation without any danger of physical injury, and cannot be used without the consent of a client's parents and the approval of a physician. Jeremy's parents had no objection to its use as a last resort on their son and no doubts concerning its safety. They had received shocks from the electric prod at their own request.

Videotapes taken by the Centre's staff showed how the cattle prod was used in Jeremy's first hour-long session. Jeremy was seated in a chair and given a jolt every time he tried to hurt himself. In that hour he managed to direct 450 blows at himself while partially restrained by members of the staff. The latter gave him verbal praise and Smarties during the brief moments when his self-abusive conduct ceased. During the first hour-long session Jeremy received 30 jolts from the cattle prod. As the aversive therapy progressed, the staff were able to decrease the number of jolts.

Within 12 months of his arrival at the Centre, Jeremy's self-destructive compulsive behaviour had been eliminated. Upon return to his home, however, he suffered a relapse. Within a month of release he was back at the Centre and treatments were resumed at the urging of Jeremy's parents. In their view, it was the only thing that would save their son from killing himself.

Question

Is using cattle prods in this way consistent with respecting Jeremy's moral dignity and worth? Or is use of a cattle prod no different, in principle, from ECT? (See Case 6:1 above.)

Case 12:2 Stephen Dawson: Should Severely Retarded Patients be Treated?

This case was first heard before Bryne, a judge of the Provincial Court of British Columbia in March, 1983 and concerned whether a simple, but life-saving surgical procedure should have been performed on Stephen Dawson, a seven-year-old boy with severe mental disabilities. Judge Bryne agreed with Stephen Dawson's parents that Stephen should be "allowed to die." The Superintendent of Family and Child Services then brought the case to The Supreme Court of British Columbia where, four days later, Mr. Justice McKenzie reversed Bryne's decision. The following description is based on the oral reasons for judgment given by the two judges.

Stephen Dawson was born prematurely on March 29, 1976 in Montreal. Shortly after his birth, Stephen suffered extensive brain damage through meningitis which inflamed the lining of his brain and left him profoundly retarded with no control over his faculties, limbs, or bodily functions. At the age of 5 months life-support surgery was performed. Surgeons implanted a plastic shunt, a tube which drains excess cerebro-spinal fluid from the head to another body cavity where it is expelled or absorbed. Without the shunt, the excess fluid would have built up in Stephen's brain, causing pain, increased incapacity and, almost certainly, eventual death.

Stephen was initially cared for at home, where he required approximately 10 hours per day of sustained care. In 1978 Stephen's family moved to British Columbia, where his parents were able to find him a place at Sunny Hill, a Vancouver institution for physically disabled children who require long term care and rehabilitation. In January of 1979 Stephen was moved to a foster home. When his parents complained, "they were told that Stephen's condition was so poor and of such low quality, that the services and facilities could be better used by others" (Bryne). Stephen remained in the foster home until February, 1982, at which point he was returned to Sunny Hill.

Stephen's parents were convinced that his life was painful and unhappy. At the hearing before Judge Bryne, the Dawsons testified that

> caring for Stephen was a full-time job. They [had] a child who [was] three years older than Stephen and another who [was] four years younger.

Stephen had to be forced to feed, forced to chew, and medication had to be forced into him. He was incontinent, regurgitated constantly, had to be fed with an eyedropper, had constant colds and respiratory problems, had seizures regularly, and could not be left alone.

Mrs. Dawson further testified that,

each feeding took two hours; that she spent eight or nine hours daily on feeding, medication, and basic needs. Plus, three hours per day for physiotherapy.

There were frequent trips to the doctor's, frequent changes in anti-epileptic medication to try to control his seizures and, further, Mr. Dawson said that bowel movements were excruciatingly painful. Stephen had a chronic nasal discharge.

Both parents testified that,

Stephen peaked when he was approximately two years old and they hoped that he was going to surpass the original diagnosis. They testified that he could hold his head up, responded to stimulation, played with the other children, could sit on a knee in the same manner as a pre-sitting baby, and they felt that he could watch T.V. even though they had been told he had been blind since the brain damage.

When the family moved to British Columbia in February 1978, Stephen caught the flu and was in and out of hospital in the spring and summer of that year. The Dawsons testified that,

the illness caused Stephen to regress. That he was in a lot of pain, that he did less and less and continued to worsen. That he ceased responding. His eyes ceased to focus, he was unaware of his surroundings, was having more seizures, and he [had] made no progress since 1978.

By the summer of 1978, Mrs. Dawson testified, she was "totally exhausted and asked for extra help from the social worker and the therapist, but they could not get any extra help, not even babysitters" (Bryne). It was at this point that the Dawsons found a place for Stephen at Sunny Hill.

Doctor Yakura, a general practitioner, testified before Judge Bryne that she had followed Stephen's progress from February 20, 1979 to February, 1982, when he was readmitted to Sunny Hill because the foster mother could not continue caring for him. She claimed,

> ... that Stephen was a passive child with profound handicaps. He was blind, had cerebral palsy, and a seizure disorder requiring multiple anti-epileptic medication three times a day and pheno-barb twice a day. He made no speech sounds and snorted from a chronic nasal discharge. She confirm[ed] the Dawsons' evidence about the difficulties in feeding him. She testified that his physical progress was no more than that of an eight-week-old infant. He would respond to pain or discomfort by moaning, fussing, or lack of appetite. With illness, his motor development would regress (Bryne).

By contrast, the professionals at Sunny Hill who had worked with Stephen over the years found him to be "a happy little fellow despite his handicaps" (McKenzie). Stephen, they urged, responded to people and smiled or laughed when stimulated. He could make sounds and giggled often. He could hold his head up, roll over from front to back, clap his hands, and reach out to operate a switch to turn on a fan or tape recorder. It was testified that he was a candidate for toilet training. The attendants who worked with Stephen found that he had been understimulated and that he had more potential than he had shown in the past.

In February of 1983, while he was at Sunny Hill, it became apparent that Stephen required a second shunt operation to repair a blockage in the shunt which, if left unattended, would have led to more brain damage, pain, and almost certainly death. The operation itself was simple and routine. Stephen's parents initially gave their consent to the remedial surgery, "but after a day's reflection, withdrew their consent on the ground that the boy should be allowed to die with dignity rather than continue to endure a life of suffering" (McKenzie). Owing to the parents' refusal to sanction the surgery, the Superintendent of Family and Child Services, acting under the provincial act which creates that office, and mindful of the provisions of that act which "make the safety and well-being of a child the paramount consideration in administering and interpreting the Act, considered this child 'in need of protection'" (McKenzie). The Superintendent presented a written report to the Provincial Court of British

Columbia asking for an order that the custody of Stephen Dawson be retained by him. Judge Bryne identified the key issue, "who may decide an incompetent's right to refuse life sustaining treatment if no directive exists and the incompetent is unable to do so?" (Bryne). She held that this legal power belongs, all else being equal, to the parents in consultation with their medical advisors. Bryne also held that where treatment would serve "only to prolong a life inflicted with an incurable condition" rather than cure or improve a patient's condition, consent to treatment may properly be withheld by parents. In her view, the shunt surgery would, in the Dawson case, constitute an "extraordinary surgical intervention." It would, in fact, "constitute cruel and unusual treatment of Stephen" (Bryne). Custody of Stephen, and with it the right to decide on his behalf, was therefore returned to the Dawsons.

Immediately following Bryne's decision, the Superintendent of Family and Child Services petitioned the Supreme Court of British Columbia for interim custody of Stephen Dawson. Mr. Justice McKenzie granted the petition, his decision being based on the following reasons.

> ... I find that the professionals who have been treating and observing Stephen since late 1982 are better qualified than [the parents] are to assess his condition and capacities because they, the parents, have hardly seen him. I do not criticize them for this but simply observe it as a fact.
>
> I cannot accept their view that Stephen would be better off dead. If it is to be decided that "it is in the best interests of Stephen Dawson that his existence cease," then it must be decided that, for him, non-existence is the better alternative. This would mean regarding the life of a handicapped child as not only less valuable than the life of a normal child, but so much less valuable that it is not worth preserving. I tremble at contemplating the consequences if the lives of disabled persons are dependent upon such judgments (McKenzie).

McKenzie ordered that temporary custody be assigned to the Superintendent of Family and Child Services and that the operation to replace the shunt be performed.

Questions

Was Judge McKenzie's decision morally defensible, or should the wishes of Stephen's parents, that the best interests of their son demanded that he be "allowed to die," have been respected? Does it matter that what they wished for was that nothing be done to prevent Stephen's death by "natural" causes? Would it have made a morally relevant difference if what they had asked for was that Stephen be given a lethal dose of morphine? If so, is this the basis upon which you would distinguish Stephen's case from the case of Tracy and her father Robert Latimer (Case 8:4)?

Case 12:3 Ought We to Save Mother or Child?

At age 22 Betty Evans's pregnancy was seriously complicated by a condition known as Eisenmenger's Complex. This condition is characterized by a hole in the partition between the right and left ventricles of the heart and a narrowing of the small arteries leading to the lung resulting in high blood pressure in the pulmonary circulation. Sufferers from Eisenmenger's Complex have very limited tolerance for exercise, experience periodic chest pains akin to angina pains associated with coronary artery disease, and periodically cough up bright red blood, due to changes in circulation in the lungs. Betty's parents did not tell her she had Eisenmenger's Complex until she was 17. When the seriousness of her condition dawned on her, and she became fully aware of the limitations imposed on her by her disease, she became quite depressed. The severity of the depression led her to make several attempts to commit suicide. She is currently very antagonistic towards her parents for failing to divulge her condition to her until she was 17, and hostile to the doctors for what she perceives as "bad management" of her case.

Because of the high risk to mother and fetus posed by Eisenmenger's Syndrome, Betty was admitted to hospital three months prior to delivery. During this period her angina-like pains and the coughing up of blood posed many problem for the cardiologists. The anaesthetists were also primed to plan appropriately for either a vaginal or a caesarian delivery. While the obstetrician pondered the risks to mother and child, the nurses and physiotherapists desperately sought to cope with a cantankerous, anxious, and sick young patient with suicidal tendencies.

In several discussions the patient was acquainted with the high risk to her life and to the life of the fetus posed by this pregnancy. The most difficult tension to be resolved focused on the mode of birth. If the woman's life were to be in jeopardy during the birth, then vaginal delivery offered better prospects for saving the mother. In case of fetal distress, a Caesarian section would be most favourable for the fetus. When these possibilities were explained to Betty and her husband, Betty was astute enough to observe that the birth could be beset by complications that would compel her care-givers to make the difficult choice of whether to save her life or the life of her child. On this the husband and wife were divided. The husband favoured saving his wife, but she was prepared to sacrifice her life to save the baby. As

Betty put it, "I have had a chance at life, my child hasn't." Remembering Betty's previous attempted suicides, her physician was worried by her expressed preference.

Question

What ought to be done if during the delivery it becomes obvious that Betty's care-givers can save her life or the baby's but not both?

Case 12:4 Should Patients be Informed of Remote Risks of Procedures?

Mr. Joe Mulroney suffered a fatal reaction to an angiogram. In the ensuing inquiry the anaesthetist admitted that he had not warned Mr. Mulroney of the remote risk of death. In fact, he did not ever warn any of his patients of the remote possibility that they might die from the procedure. In his view, and in the view of the majority of his colleagues, death in such circumstances was rare enough that to mention it would unduly alarm patients. Indeed, at the hospital at which that angiogram was done on Mr. Mulroney, they had an excellent track record. Over five thousand angiograms had been done there over a decade without a single fatality.

Sean, Mr. Mulroney's son, unimpressed by such statistics, insisted his father should have been told of the risk of death. "Surely," he argued, "that's what informed consent is all about."

The anaesthetist then raised the question whether it would have made any material difference to the case if Mr. Mulroney had been informed. "Do you really think he would have refused the procedure if I had explained the odds to him? He struck me as being a very reasonable man and most reasonable people choose the angiogram. So why burden your father or others with information that might only present a problem for a small or even a nonexistent minority? Surely giving full information in this case would be counter to the patient's best interests."

"That is a value judgment rather than a medical judgment," Joe's son retorted. Many patients would consider it in their best interests to know all the risks involved in a given procedure and I happen to be one of those people. Only a paternalist who shows lack of respect for patients as persons would think or act otherwise. You should not have assumed that my father would have opted for the procedure. Even if your assumption is correct, and if it should turn out from future studies that the majority of patients would also choose the procedure, they – not their care-givers – should make the choice."

"I beg to differ," responded the anaesthetist. "One has to consider the burden of fear and distress placed on patients when informing them of harms with an extremely low probability factor."

"Low probability factor or not," replied the son, "patients have a right to be given full information about any procedure to which they are subjected. While I do not hold you responsible for my father's death, I think you were delinquent in your duty as a practitioner in failing to apprise him of the risk involved, however remote. While there might be rare exceptions to informing patients about remote risks, the practice of not informing them is morally indefensible."

Question

Who is right? Joe's son or the anaesthetist?

Case 12:5 Whistle Blowing on Hepatitis B Carriers

Marjorie Williams, a 25-year-old woman, visited her physician complaining of nausea, feverishness, persistent tiredness, and abdominal pains. The test for hepatitis B surface antigen turned out to be positive. When questioned by her physician about her sexual life, she admitted to having several sexual partners. Concern about the danger of her infecting her sexual partners prompted the physician to propose that she inform them about the results of the test. She refused to comply with the proposal on the grounds that the presence of hepatitis B antigen does not necessarily indicate that she actually is infectious. The physician agreed that while essentially true, this observation overlooks the fact that there is some evidence for the sexual transmission of hepatitis B by "asymptomatic carriers." So if she were to persist in her sexual activity, her physician would feel a strong obligation to report her case to the appropriate authorities. At this Marjorie stormed out of the doctor's office, muttering accusations about breach of patient confidentiality.

Question

What should the doctor do in this case – maintain confidentiality or report Marjorie to the appropriate authority?

Case 12:6 Minors as Organ Donors

Nancy was a 10-year-old profoundly retarded child who had been institutionalized from birth. She suffered from end-stage renal failure. A kidney transplant was recommended as the treatment of choice. Over the years, Sylvia and Jack, Nancy's parents, not only had formed a deep affection for Nancy, but had been very supportive of her. It came as no surprise, therefore, that both volunteered to donate a kidney for transplantation in an effort to save her life. Because of tissue incompatibility both offers had to be rejected. Tests done on Olive, Nancy's 12-year-old sister confirmed her to be a potential donor. Furthermore, Olive expressed a willingness to respond to her sister's need. This generous gesture, as far as could be determined, was just that, and was neither the product of coercion nor prompted by a pathological affection for her sister. On the contrary, the affection for her sister appeared to be quite genuine.

In deep distress the parents turned to Jack's brother, Harry, for counsel. It is moot whether Harry was a hindrance rather than a help. He was strongly against allowing Olive to donate a kidney to Nancy. Since Olive was a minor, her parents were required to sign the consent form for surgery. Harry made no bones about insisting that they would be delinquent in their duty as parents if they were to place their healthy daughter at risk for the sake of their younger, profoundly retarded, child.

Sylvia and Jack were greatly taken aback by this onslaught. How could Harry so quickly dismiss the idea that the strong should be allowed to volunteer to come to the rescue of the weak? "Think of the message we shall be sending out to handicapped children everywhere if we take what you say seriously. You surely would not want to generalize your reticence to place the healthy at risk for the unhealthy. Surely assuming such a risk is a part of what's involved in bearing one another's burdens."

Unimpressed, Harry replied, "Please don't get religious on me with your appeals to bear one another's burdens."

"But I'm not meaning to sound religious about this," Sylvia retorted. "I think a good humanist would argue the same way."

"If by a good humanist you mean someone who approaches problems rationally, then I think a humanist would agree with me," countered Harry. "I would like to resolve this conflict by appealing to reason rather than to emotion. While my heart is with you, my head tells me that it is unreasonable to put the healthy at risk to protect the weak. Even if Olive were an adult, she would have no obligation to donate an organ to another, no matter how great that other person's need. Organ donation is a work of supererogation rather than of obligation. Since, however, Olive is only a minor, she needs to be protected against having a decision made for her she might later regret. As her parents and guardians you may not project your own charitable inclinations on your daughter. It is your duty to protect her."

Questions

What ought the parents to do in this case? Does Harry have a point when he suggests that donating an organ to a sibling who requires it to survive is not obligatory but rather supererogatory, that is, beyond the call of moral duty? Assuming that Olive's wishes are genuine, is it appropriate for her parents to exercise their right to make surrogate decisions on her behalf by honouring her wishes? Bear in mind that she is only 12 years of age. Can she fully appreciate the nature and consequences of her heroic offer? If Olive's wishes should not be determinative, and any surrogate decision must be based instead on Olive's best interests, is it possible that those interests lie in helping her sister? Consider whether any of your answers to the preceding questions would change if Nancy were *not* profoundly disabled? Once you have done so, test your moral judgments against the issues raised in the following case.

Case 12:7 Failed Contraception, Genetic Defect, and Parental Disagreement

At 36 years of age Betsy discovered she was pregnant for the third time. Her pregnancy, the result of failed contraception, took her and her husband by surprise. Neither Betsy nor Bill favoured abortion. However, in view of her age, and since there was a history of Down's syndrome in the family, Betsy requested that an amniocentesis be done at the appropriate time to determine the health status of her child. She expressed a willingness to continue the pregnancy to term provided the results of the amniocentesis were negative. Otherwise she would seek a therapeutic abortion.

Bill had great difficulty in accepting this. He objected, "Failed contraception and handicap do not add up to compelling reasons for seeking an abortion." He then went on to elaborate, "It is one thing to use contraceptive measures to prevent conception, quite another thing to use abortion as a back-up for contraceptive failure. Is that not exactly what we would be doing if we sought an abortion should the test prove to be positive? Added to that, would we not be seeking an abortion for the wrong reason? Would we not be terminating the pregnancy because our child is handicapped? Think of the message our action would send out to the handicapped – that non-existence is preferable to handicapped existence. It's not as though we can tell in advance whether our Down's child will be mildly or profoundly retarded. Since we can't be sure of this, I feel strongly that such a child should be given the benefit of the doubt. After all, Down's children are not only capable of giving and receiving affection, and leading rewarding lives, they are also adoptable."

To this Betsy could only reply, "I understand what you are saying, Bill. But I honestly don't think I can cope with a disabled child. I am as disappointed in myself as you must be with me. But that's the way I am and that's how I feel."

Reluctantly, Bill responded, "Since you feel that strongly about it, I will try to support you in your decision."

At eighteen weeks, amniocentesis revealed Betsy to be carrying an afflicted fetus, whereupon she requested an abortion. With this request the seriousness of Bill's misgivings came to the fore. He had hoped against hope that the results of the amniocentesis would have been negative. He had pledged to support Betsy, but now that the time had come he found it very difficult to follow through on his pledge.

Both he and Betsy were visibly shaken by the results. Though very upset, Betsy reiterated her request for an abortion. The prospect of having a Downs child terrified her. She felt utterly unequipped to care for a disabled child. She also believed that having such a child would place undue strain on her marriage and would be terribly unfair to their other two children, Harry, 10 years old and Monica, 7 years old. Bill, however, still could not rid himself of the conviction that to abort their disabled child would be tantamount to shirking their responsibility. He insisted, "We owe this child a chance at life. After all, if it gets too much for us, we can consider placing the child in an institution. But let's not make that decision until we at least give it a try."

Nonplussed by this turn of events, the physician sought the opinion of members of the Ethics Discussion Service.

Questions

Imagine that you are a member of an Ethics Discussion Service. What would you advise the physician to do? Might it be different from what you think the parents ought to do?

Case 12:8 Sex Selection For Non-Medical Reasons

Jackie and Tom Simpson were a happily married couple with three children, Sally, Janie, and Donna. Jackie and Tom were both 28 years of age, while Sally was 9, Janie 6, and Donna 2. Though he loved his three girls, Tom very much wanted a son with whom he could share certain of his interests, such as team sports, fishing, and camping. He also thought it important that, as an only child, he have a son of his own to carry on the family name. When it became known that Jackie was in her second month of pregnancy, Jackie indicated her willingness to have a prenatal diagnostic procedure performed which would reveal the sex of her fetus. If it turned out that the fetus was female, she would be willing to undergo a therapeutic abortion following which they could try again for a boy. She knew how important it was to Tom that he have a son. If on the other hand, the fetus was male, then Jackie would allow the pregnancy to proceed to term. She noted that modern prenatal diagnostic techniques have developed to the point where they are virtually risk-free for both the woman and her fetus. She also noted that a local fertility clinic routinely provides prenatal testing services for pregnant women who, for reasons of age or family history, are at risk of having severely disabled children.

When the Simpsons met with the staff at the fertility clinic, they were told in no uncertain terms that what they were proposing was highly unethical. Under no circumstances were the staff at the clinic prepared to perform such a procedure for the purposes the Simpsons had in mind. Sex selection for non-medical reasons reinforces the idea that the sex of a child is important, and encourages the view that families with all boys or all girls are less than ideal. Furthermore, it could make Sally, Janie, and Donna feel that their own sex was lacking in some way, and would only serve to reinforce sexual stereotypes which work to the detriment of women. What's to prevent Tom from sharing his interests in team sports, fishing, and camping with his daughters? Nothing. Prenatal diagnosis for purposes of sex selection is an immoral and wasteful use of scarce resources.

Questions

Is it immoral to allow prenatal diagnosis for the purposes the Simpsons have in mind? Was the Simpson's wish based on prejudice? Or can it be rational and moral to want a child of a particular sex for the types of reasons Tom has articulated? Suppose that Jackie were 38 years of age and therefore entitled, because hers was a high-risk pregnancy, to the prenatal diagnosis. If the procedure were done, and revealed Jackie to be carrying a female fetus, would she then be justified in aborting the fetus to try again for a boy? If they knew her intentions, would the staff of the fertility clinic have been justified in withholding information about the sex of a fetus which the tests had determined to be fully normal?

Case 12:9 To Resuscitate or Not to Resuscitate?

At 89, Sam Levinworth was admitted to hospital with bronchial pneumonia, advanced pulmonary edema (fluid in the lungs), and urinary tract infection. It so happened that the hospital was experimenting with a new admission form calculated to determine patients' wishes about their future care. When the question of cardiopulmonary resuscitation was raised Sam responded by saying, "If my heart stops beating, just get it going again." Jenny, Sam's wife, agreed with her husband's request. From gentle probing to ensure valid consent, it was uncertain whether either of them fully understood what was involved in the procedure, or of its low success rate with elderly patients. Cardiopulmonary resuscitation consists of one or all of the following procedures: chest compressions, artificial respiration, intubation, ventilation, defibrillation, and pacing.

Although the physician had misgivings about acquiescing in their request he promised to respect their wishes. The nurses were less than enamoured of what they considered to be an unreasonable and unrealistic capitulation to patient's wishes. They advocated another round of negotiations with Sam and his wife in an attempt to convince them that the right to treatment did not include the right to useless treatment. The physician, however, decided to adopt a wait-and-see-what-happens attitude.

After ten days in hospital Sam was responding poorly to treatment. His prognosis was dismal and in the words of the physician, "Sam's vital processes just seem to be shutting down." Nurse Williams then asked, "What do we do if he arrests?"

"I don't know," replied the physician. "Let's talk to his wife."

After raising the question of CPR with her, Jenny insisted she still wanted "everything done for Sam, including CPR." When the physician proposed talking again to Sam, Jenny became quite agitated and said, "Don't harass my husband with such a sensitive question at a time like this. It would give him the wrong message. How can you ask, "Do you want to be resuscitated?" without making it sound like a rhetorical question that invites 'No' for an answer? I won't let you do that to him. He already expressed his wish about CPR ten days ago. He was more lucid then than now. So I think we should go with his earlier decision."

"But," replied the physician, "his condition was not as serious then as now. If he knew of his hopeless prognosis, do you think he would still have wanted CPR?"

To which Mrs. Levinworth replied, "Where there's life there's hope."

At that moment a nurse came running out of Sam's room crying, "Sam's stopped breathing and there are no vital signs. What do you want me to do?"

Questions

What should the physician do? Bow to Jenny's and Sam's wishes? Or should she act on the basis of her best medical judgment and refuse to resuscitate Sam? Would it have made any difference if it was clear that both Jenny and Sam fully understood what was involved in CPR, and that it is pointless in Sam's case? What if Sam were revived but entered a coma from which he never recovered? Would the hard decisions simply have been postponed? Is it relevant that vital scarce resources would then be used to sustain Sam when they might have been used to help patients for whom they might have provided some benefit?

Case 12:10 CPR and a Nurse's Responsibility (1)

Stella was a highly skilled and knowledgeable critical-care nurse with 25 years of experience in the ICU. Sally was a 76-year-old woman suffering from an incurable brain tumour. Informed opinion was that Sally would likely die within two weeks.

With Sally's consent, a DNR (Do-not-resuscitate) order had been placed on her chart. This meant that Sally would not be resuscitated should she experience cardiac arrest.

One afternoon, while Stella was working in the ICU, Sally grabbed her arm. Sally was partially conscious and began mumbling, "I don't want to die. Please don't let me die." Following this brief period of partial lucidity, Sally lapsed again into unconsciousness after which point she quickly began to arrest. Instinctively, Stella started to call for help in resuscitating Sally, but pulled back when she remembered the DNR order. She let the arrest take its course and Sally quickly died. Stella was very uneasy about what she had done, but came to terms with her decision for the following reasons. (1) Resuscitation was not in Sally's best interests; (2) a valid DNR order had been issued; and (3) despite her (questionable) mumbling, Sally had earlier agreed that CPR would not be in her best interests.

Questions

Was Stella right in dismissing Sally's mumblings? Should we perhaps always err on the side of caution in cases such as these? Should we always resuscitate if there is any question about the patient's continued consent to a DNR order, even if resuscitation continues to be futile?

Case 12:11 CPR and a Nurse's Responsibility (2)

Stella was a highly skilled and knowledgeable critical-care nurse with 25 years of experience in the ICU. Sally was an intermittently conscious, 76-year-old woman suffering from an incurable brain tumour. Informed opinion was that Sally would likely die within two weeks.

Sally's physician, Dr. Allen, sought informed consent for a DNR (Do-not-resuscitate) order. Such an order would mean that Sally would not be resuscitated should she experience cardiac arrest. Despite agreement that her situation was hopeless and that she was at the end of her life, Sally wished to be resuscitated should she suffer cardiac arrest. "Life is life," she said.

One afternoon, while Stella was doing her rounds in the ICU, Sally grabbed Stella's arm. She was fully conscious and said, "I've changed my mind. I don't want you to do CPR on me if I arrest. I've had a good, long life and nothing would be gained by bringing me back." Stella said, "Are you sure about this?" to which Sally replied, "I'm as sure of this as I've ever been sure of anything." "All right," replied Stella, "I'll have a talk with Dr. Allen. I'm sure he will agree to issue the order."

As Stella was leaving to find Dr. Allen, Sally began to arrest. Instinctively, Stella started to call for help in resuscitating Sally, but pulled back when she remembered the conversation she had just had with Sally. Instead she held Sally's hand while she died.

Questions

Was Stella's omission morally justified? Or was she obliged to resuscitate given that there was no DNR order? Did it matter that Sally had changed her mind and requested that such an order be given? Did it matter that Dr. Allen had earlier attempted to get consent for such an order? Would it have mattered if the hospital had a policy requiring that patients always be resuscitated by nursing staff unless there is a valid DNR order on the patient's chart signed by a physician? Would such a policy violate patient autonomy? Would such a policy be an affront to the moral and professional integrity of nurses such as Stella, whose knowledge, expertise, and intimate contact with patients often place them in an ideal position to make such difficult life-and-death decisions on behalf of their patients?

Case 12:12 "Please Don't Tell My Husband He Has Cancer"

In his seventieth year Jay McMurtry was referred by his family doctor to a urologist with a tentative diagnosis of carcinoma of the prostate gland. Surgery confirmed the diagnosis. Immediately following the operation, while Jay was still in intensive care, the surgeon met with Mrs. McMurtry and her son, Jim. Anxiously, Mrs. McMurtry inquired about the outcome of the surgery. The surgeon was truthful but sensitive in informing the patient's wife and son that the diagnosis had been confirmed. Jay McMurtry had cancer of the prostate gland.

Tearfully, both Mrs. McMurtry and her son pleaded with the surgeon to withhold this bad news from Jay. She explained, "Jay has always been a nervous man, and prone to periods of depression. Emotionally he is not very robust." She then went on to explain that her husband had been very worried about himself from the moment surgery was proposed. The worry was no doubt intensified by the fact that he had lost a close friend about a year ago to prostatic carcinoma. For this reason, she added, he will, doubtless, envisage a parallel fate for himself if he discovers that he has cancer of the prostate gland. Mrs. McMurtry then went on to say, "I don't think he will be able to handle the truth about his condition. At least, not right now."

By way of reply, the surgeon related how in his experience patients were much more capable of handling the truth than their family members gave them credit for. Anyway, would it not show a lack of respect towards Jay to treat him in this paternalistic way?

"I don't think so," said Mrs. McMurtry. "But even if it did, I still think his well-being is more important to him and to us than the satisfaction of having been told 'the truth, the whole truth, and nothing but the truth.' Do you understand what I am saying, doctor?"

"I think I do," replied the surgeon. "While I have some reservations, I will do as you ask."

"Thank you," said Mrs. McMurtry. "One more thing, doctor; please do not say anything meanwhile to our family physician." Obviously taken aback, the physician responded, "You are asking a lot of me, Mrs McMurtry. First you ask me to withhold the truth from your husband, and now you ask me to withhold information from a colleague."

To this Mrs. McMurtry retorted, "If you tell our family physician, you might as well tell my husband."

"Are you sure of that?" inquired the surgeon.

"I've never been more sure of anything in my life," was the reply. "So, please, do me a favour, either tell neither or tell both of them. Needless to say, I would prefer that you tell neither."

After thinking it over for a few moments, the surgeon said, "I will respect your wishes, Mrs. McMurtry, and tell neither."

Questions

Did the surgeon behave ethically in acquiescing to Mrs. McMurtry's double barrelled request? Is it ever right to withhold important information from competent patients on grounds of "their best interests"? Or is such paternalistically motivated action always an unwarranted affront to human dignity? Is it a violation of both professional and moral duty not to tell the patient's family physician under such circumstances?

Case 12:13 "Don't Start the Respirator"

At age 10 Bernice Kinsley was involved in a car accident. She was admitted to hospital with what appeared to be superficial head injuries. While Bernice had suffered a concussion, X-rays had revealed no fractures. She appeared to be quite chipper when her parents left the hospital that night.

At 3:00 a.m., while making a routine bed check, Nurse Wilson noticed that Bernice's skin was blue and that she was not breathing. Her pupils were fixed and dilated. Nurse Wilson set the machinery in motion for cardiopulmonary resuscitation, CPR.

With the help of the resident, Bernice was intubated, hooked to a cardiac monitor, and given appropriate drug therapy. After forty minutes a heartbeat was restored, but her pupils were still fixed and dilated. The signs were not good. The resident suspected that Bernice's brain had been deprived of oxygen to the point where irreversible damage had been done. Nurse Wilson then proposed that Bernice be placed on a respirator in the ICU. This would enable Bernice's caregivers to test at intervals to determine with greater certainty whether or not she was brain dead.

The resident appeared to be very uncomfortable with this suggestion. He said, "Once we put her on the respirator we will be forced to continue treatment. Would it not be easier on the parents, the family, and us if we didn't start the machine? I honestly believe that she's too far gone to come back to us."

Nurse Wilson objected strenuously to the resident's proposal. "We can't be sure," she said, "that Bernice is beyond our power to help her. We must at least try. If after two tests she has a flat electroencephalogram then we can turn off the machine."

With serious misgivings the resident concurred with Nurse Wilson's wishes.

Questions

Did the resident do the right thing in acquiescing to Nurse Wilson's suggestion? Or should he have based his decision on his medical judgment and resisted putting Bernice on the respirator? Would it have made a difference to that judgment to learn that Bernice continued to breathe on her own, but is still comatose ten months later?

Case 12:14 Queue-Jumping in the OR

Mrs. Susan Darling is a 43-year-old mother of two, who is also married to a physician. Her general health is good except for a mild anxiety disorder. As part of her regular health care examination, Susan had a screening mammogram. This revealed a small lump in the left breast.

Susan's physician, Dr. White, arranged for her to see a general surgeon who did an excisional biopsy. This revealed the lump to be a low-grade malignancy.

Following this discovery, Dr. White booked Susan for an elective lumpectomy with an axillary node exploration. Given the nature of the case, he booked the operation on his regular operating room time for two weeks hence. Dr. White had many more urgent cases which he had decided to book before Susan's.

Susan's husband, Dr. Darling, called Dr. White to see if the case could be moved up. Dr. White told him that this was the next available time for a case of this urgency.

Dr. Darling did not end the matter here. He next contacted the OR Director to see if there was an earlier time in which the operation could be performed by someone else. The Director noted that there was time available in Dr. Black's schedule which was presently unbooked. Without telling Dr. White, the OR Director arranged for the operation to be performed in three days. An anxiety disorder was cited as the official reason to change the timing of the operation.

Questions

Was it morally correct for Dr. Darling to attempt to jump the queue in the way that he did? By exerting pressure on a colleague to do him a personal favour did he exploit his position? Was it right for the OR Director to facilitate Dr. Darling's request when he would in all likelihood have turned down a member of the general public? Would this be unjust? Or is this the kind of case where the personal ties so crucial to moral life must be allowed to sway the decision in favour of a friend and colleague? Finally, was it right for Dr. Darling and the Director to make the decisions they did without consulting Dr. White?

Case 12:15 An "Over-the-Hill" Surgeon

Dr. Blake is a 60-year-old surgeon. His technical skills are not what they used to be. In addition, there has been a plethora of recent advances in operating techniques with which Dr. Blake has not been able to keep abreast. The result is that Dr. Blake is now experiencing a great many technical difficulties. His judgment is as good as ever, however, and on occasion he realizes that help is needed for which he is not afraid to ask.

Despite his conscientiousness and willingness to seek assistance when necessary, Dr. Blake is taking more and longer time to finish routine cases. Recently, a case which normally should take thirty minutes took longer than two full hours. This was caused by Dr. Blake's inability to deal adequately with a technical problem which his colleagues could have dealt with quickly and efficiently. The difficulty was dealt with, but not without undue stress caused to Dr. Blake and the OR attendants, and increased risk to the patient.

A further consequence of Dr. Blake's inability to operate efficiently is that the case ran overtime, causing the cancellation of another case. The cancelled patient was brought back the next day and again Dr. Blake took longer than normal, resulting in the OR running overtime for a second time.

Both the anaesthetist and the circulating nurse are greatly concerned, but neither is sure how to proceed. Patient risk is a grey area, and the inefficient utilization of scare resources is another. On the other hand, Dr. Blake is personable, eloquent, a fine member of the community with a long and distinguished career.

Questions

Do their concerns morally warrant the anaesthetist and the circulating nurse in approaching the OR Director with the problem of Dr. Blake's inefficiency and its attendant risks? If he were approached, what should the OR Director do? How does personal loyalty, and the feelings of a hard-working, conscientious surgeon stack up against increased risk to patients and the inefficient use of a scarce resource like OR time?

index